Unlock Autism

7-Step Autism Action Plan™ to
Unlock Your Child's Potential
Within 12 Months

Unlock Autism
7-Step Autism Action Plan™ to Unlock Your Child's Potential Within 12 Months
© 2024 Taiba Bajar

ISBN: 9781068620102 Paperback

Published by: Inspired By Publishing

Cover Design by: Tanya Grant – The TNG Designs Group Limited

The strategies in this book are presented primarily for enjoyment and educational purposes. Every effort has been made to trace copyright holders and obtain their permission for the use of copyright material.

The information and resources provided in this book are based upon the authors' personal experiences. Any outcome, income statements or other results, are based on the authors' experiences and there is no guarantee that your experience will be the same. There is an inherent risk in any business enterprise or activity and there is no guarantee that you will have similar results as the author as a result of reading this book.

The author reserves the right to make changes and assumes no responsibility or liability whatsoever on behalf of any purchaser or reader of these materials.

Disclaimer: I want to make it clear that I am not a doctor. This book is for educational purposes only and should not be seen as medical advice. All client names in this book have been changed for confidentiality. At the time of publishing I am not affiliated with any of the brands or products mentioned in this book.

Acknowledgements

To my amazing parents, Sharif Bajar and Muzammal Bajar. I am so thankful for your love, sacrifices and unlimited support. Your selflessness and dedication have opened countless doors of opportunity for me and my siblings and have shaped me into the person I am today. You are my role models, my inspiration, and I am forever grateful for being born to such amazing parents. Throughout my own journey of parenthood, I am so blessed to have you as shining examples. Thank you for everything; you are my heroes.

To my husband Shehroz Mushtaq. Your non-stop love and support for me since the day we got married has been amazing. Your constant love has actually built up my self esteem and self belief so much and I am so grateful to have you as my husband. My best friend and partner for life inshallah.

To all of my siblings, Imran, Lubna, Saymah, Ehsaan, and especially Uzma and Sidrah. Being one of seven children is quite a life defining experience. All of my siblings, and especially Uzma and Sidrah, have been non-stop supporters of my career goals and family goals, and I really appreciate having you in my corner. Thank you.

To all of my aunties, uncles, cousins, nieces and nephews. You've all been there for me consistently in my life, and I don't take that for granted at all. Especially Akram Bajar, Ashraf Bajar, Yasmin Bajar and Fouzia Bajar.

To my best friends, Dr Salma Aslam and Dr Javariah Jabbar. You are both the definition of supportive best friends, taught me how to be strong, to stand up for myself and are my constant companions. I couldn't have asked for better friends and I am so grateful for having you both in my life and for your constant encouragement, support, belief and love.

To my two wonderful children, thank you for letting me be your Mum. I love watching you both grow.

To Shalah Akhtar, who helped me believe in myself and has encouraged me non-stop.

To Shahroo Izadi, whose book *The Kindness Method* changed my life, changed the self-talk in my mind and gave me the confidence to achieve things I never thought possible and to believe in myself.

To Chloë Bisson for her amazing book, *Just Write The Damn Book*, which was a massive inspiration and kick up the bum for me to write this book.

Contents

Introduction

Why You Need to Read This Book!

If you're reading this book, it's likely because your child or a loved one's child has an autism diagnosis. Or if you're in the UK like me, you might be suspecting autism in your child, but are still waiting for your child's official diagnosis.

I remember how overwhelming and emotional this experience can be. You may have turned to your GP or Health Visitor for help, but perhaps you didn't receive the support you hoped for. If you're fortunate enough not to have been dismissed, your child may have been placed on a waiting list for assessment, which determines their access to services. Following the assessment, there's often another waiting list for the actual support to begin. This system can be frustrating, and unfortunately, there's often insufficient support available for parents of autistic children in our country. Even after receiving an official diagnosis, some parents still struggle to access the help their child needs, leaving them feeling like they're left to manage everything on their own.

Within the autism community I found that there are two main types of narratives. There are people who will try to convince you that "this is a lifelong condition that your child is born with. Their brain is wired like this, and there is nothing you can do except adapt your child's environment in a loving way to try and make their life experiences easier for them." This is the narrative I was told. I was told to look for a SEN school, purchase noise cancelling headphones for my child, and be prepared to look after a child who may never become independent or will always have some lifelong struggles.

I couldn't accept this narrative, and if you're reading this book, I'm sure you feel the same way and you are looking for solutions to unlock the potential you see within your child.

There is a second more hopeful emerging narrative that a person's brain can be rewired. Neuroplasticity is the name given for the ability to create new brain connections and reorganise and prune your old brain connections. Understanding neuroplasticity means understanding that there is the potential to change the brain you currently have or the brain you are born with. When you've done this, you can change your habits and learn new skills. As parents this means we can help rewire our autistic children's brains, help them to thrive in new environments and adapt to sensory changes better, and to learn new skills faster such as speech, emotional intelligence, and potty training.

Thankfully I remembered learning about the potential of the brain, especially how malleable a child's brain is in the first five years of their life from my neuroscience studies at university. A child's brain has grown 75% of the brain connections it will ever have by the age of 3, and would have grown by 90% of the brain connections by age 5.[1] Even after this age of rapid physical growth, there is evidence of neuroplasticity occurring even in adults up until the age of 75, and as more research happens, it is likely that we will discover evidence of neuroplasticity occurring beyond this age too. So if your autistic child is older than the age of 5, there is still a lot of potential to use neuroplasticity to rewire their brain, overcome any developmental delays, and unlock their potential.

Sometimes it can be difficult to know if our child really does have autism. Or are they just developing a bit slower than normal? Use "Worksheet: How Do I Know If My Child Even Has Autism?" on page 17 to help you answer this question for yourself. As parents, we are often first to see autism symptoms in our children below the age of 3-5. Because of how fast the brain grows in this age, this also means there is a lot we can do to influence our child's life outcomes at this age.

When a person's inputs change, e.g. their nutrition, their stress levels, the toxins they are exposed to, their hormone levels, their environment etc., then this changes the outputs (symptoms) they display. This can be regardless of what genes they have. A person's genes are not their destiny. The environment has an impact on the expression of genes. For example, a person could have a gene for obesity, but if they are living in an environment where there are a lot of food shortages or they have a healthy lifestyle where they are staying fit and not overeating, then that person will never show that gene's expression of being obese. This is what epigenetics teaches us. How having the gene for something does not make it a person's destiny, but that gene expressions can be switched on or off depending on the person's environment and lifestyle.

In the case of an autistic child who is experiencing a developmental delay and showing autism symptoms, which are impacting the quality of their life and their family's lives, I will be teaching you my 7-Step Autism Action Plan™. This is a step-by-step guide on how to change each of your child's inputs to produce different outcomes for them: someone who may no longer have sensory overwhelm or underwhelm; someone who is no longer always so anxious or aggressive; someone who reaches their developmental milestones; or someone whose potential has now been unlocked, who can lead themselves *and* others.

I have included some worksheets throughout this book to guide you on how to implement the 7-Step Autism Action Plan for your child. If you follow my step-by-step method, your child will likely make progress towards their developmental milestones and you will know exactly how to unlock their potential within 12 months. As a parent, I know that after seeing nil or limited developmental progress in your child, I know that this is a bold promise. But it is one that I know can be fulfilled as I have done this for my own son, and for many of my clients' autistic children too. My program works. Everyone can rewire their brains to learn new skills using neuroplasticity, if they optimise their brain health by changing the inputs their brain is receiving.[2]

Autism is not simply in a child's genes where there is nothing you can do about it. Research conducted by Professor John Constantino, of psychiatry and pediatrics at Washington University studied identical twins who had an official autism diagnosis. He explained that autism severity often varies greatly between identical twins. For example, one twin could be non-verbal and the other could have excellent speech. This shows that the quality of life of autistic children is not hardwired by their genetics.[3] It proves that the environment matters a lot, which should be hopeful to us parents as it shows even if a child has a strong genetic vulnerability to display autism symptoms, there's a lot of room for improvement to reduce their symptoms and enhance their quality of life.

Before I go any further, I want to make it clear that at the age of 23, I discovered that I was on the autism spectrum and I also received a diagnosis of dyspraxia. Once I got my diagnoses, this made a lot of sense, as there were always skills that I found harder to learn and social situations where I didn't understand nuances as well as other people. However sadly, once I learned my labels, I leaned into them harder and limited myself. As an example, I always enjoyed learning Bollywood choreography dances growing up. As soon as I learned that I had dyspraxia, I accepted that "this will be harder for me and I won't be able to get this skill easily." I believed that I would find this skill harder to learn so I tried less, and my dance moves got worse, and my confidence to perform in front of other people decreased. Sadly this is similar for my team working skills, or my social skills at events or to form new friendship groups as adults. I only wish I discovered neuroplasticity earlier at 18, and I wouldn't have limited myself so much in my twenties. Also, once I started adopting the lifestyle change that I implemented for my son, my own autism symptoms mostly disappeared too.

Labels can help a person understand themselves better, but as parents, we don't want to add a label to our child's self-image so that it becomes a self-fulfilling prophecy, and they struggle more in those areas.

In the 1960s, psychologist Howard Becker talked about the "labelling theory,"[4] saying that the labels society gives us affect how we act. This idea means that labels can become like predictions, influencing what we do. You may have seen this in your own life. For example, after a series of not-so-great friendships, you may label yourself as "not likeable." You may perform badly on one math test and label yourself as "not very good at math." Or missing one timely opportunity and you may label yourself as "not proactive." The important thing to know is that labels can cut the other way. Bad labels can make behaviours worse, but good labels can make them better.

Personally, when I'm feeling unsure about myself, I like to label myself "lifelong learner." This positive label shows how I'm determined to move forward, keep learning, and applying what I learned. It helps me focus on learning from challenges and moving forward rather than getting stuck on what went wrong. A "lifelong learner" keeps reflecting and moving forward, they wouldn't let setbacks stop them for long. Labels are like tools that shape how we see ourselves. If we change our labels, we can often change how we act.

For autistic individuals, there is an understanding that they will find relationships skills and social situations harder throughout their lives. Robert Waldinger's famous Ted talk "What Makes A Good Life? Lessons From The Longest Study On Happiness" makes it clear from his 85-year study (and still counting) that the strength of a person's social connections has the biggest impact on the strength of their physical and mental health throughout their lives. I didn't want my son to realise he had the label of "autism," and self-fulfil the prophecy that he was going to find relationships and social connections harder. And, based on Robert Waldinger's study, this sets him up for worse physical and mental health throughout his lifetime. At the time, I found it challenging to strike a balance. I wanted others to understand my child's struggles with autism, rather than simply seeing him as misbehaving. I also aimed to provide him with the support he needed to thrive, while ensuring he maintained a strong sense of self as an individual capable of achieving anything with determination.

I also want to make it clear that there is nothing wrong with the label autism. I have an autism diagnosis, and I'm the mother of a son who is on the autism spectrum. But the families I work with often struggle with children who are so stressed that they are scratching themselves in social situations; who are older than the age of four but still aren't potty trained; who have such a limited diet that they suffer from nutritional deficiencies; or who are non-verbal or suffer from anxiety, and so are selectively mute. Autistic individuals can also suffer from anxiety or aggressive tendencies, and are at four times greater risk of having mental health conditions (including depression, anxiety, and bipolar syndrome) as adults.[5] Even after getting an official diagnosis in this country, families are often left to deal with everything themselves, with very little interventional support.

As a parent, I dreamed of my child having a life where he can thrive in every situation, can live independently, and lead himself and others into the life he dreams of. I saw it as my responsibility to learn as much as I could about autism and brain development to ensure that my child doesn't struggle throughout his life, doesn't battle any mental health condition he is statistically more likely to get, and that he doesn't become an adult who hasn't been able to fulfil his potential—which ultimately means he isn't able to enjoy life as much as he could. So I learned everything I could to help my child have more choices in his life as an adult, to help him choose to live any life that he wanted. If you're reading this book, I'm sure you wish the same for your autistic child / children too.

I also want to make it clear that my 7-Step Autism Action Plan to unlock your child's potential is different from "masking," which some autistic children (especially girls) may do. Masking is when autistic individuals hide their traits,[6] like stimming or avoiding eye contact in social situations, only to have meltdowns and depressive episodes later when they're alone. The 7-Step Autism Action Plan doesn't involve teaching new behaviours through therapies like ABA therapy. Instead, it focuses on addressing the biological reasons behind their symptoms. For example, fixing a leaky gut, reducing toxin levels, or helping the cerebellum grow to a normal size. This way you can unlock your child's potential and they can learn new skills faster, overcoming any developmental delays they may have.

Mitochondrial Theory of Autism

Often as humans, we like to think of one source causing one effect. Cause and Effect. Very simple to understand. In real life, this isn't actually the case. For autism, there has been such a wide range of popular theories that pinpoint a particular cause of autism.

Is it environmental toxins or infections the mother had while she was pregnant? Is it exposure to general anaesthetic, dietary patterns of the parents and child, exposure to drugs while in the womb or even vaccinations which causes the child to show autism symptoms? There is something that links all of those possible causes together, which is that they all affect the mitochondrial biology of the child.

Mitochondria are often called the powerhouse of a cell. Mitochondria is a structure which is in almost every cell of the human body. It most famously makes ATP, which is the molecule used for energy. However mitochondria also have a wide range of other important functions. This includes sending signals between other cells, maintaining the balance of ions in a cell,[7] and they are also involved in the production and regulation of reactive oxygen species in a cell and more.[8]

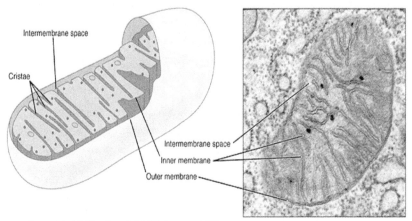

Annotated Mitochondria: Picture and Diagram.
This picture is from: Zuryn, S. (2017) *Mitochondria: What are they and why do we have them?*, *Queensland Brain Institute - University of Queensland* [9]

Think of your body as a house, and the mitochondria are like the power source keeping everything running smoothly. The mitochondrial theory of autism suggests that if there's a problem with this power source, it could lead to conditions like autism spectrum disorder, bipolar disorder, or depression. Scientists have been discussing this theory since 1986. They have also found evidence in people with autism and mitochondrial disease that supports this idea, like unusual chemical patterns and signs of inflammation in a person with autism.[10]

Dr. Chris Palmer is a Harvard University Professor and Psychiatrist. In his 2022 book "Brain Energy," he directly relates the role of mitochondria underlying the expression of all brain disorders (autism, ADHD, bipolar disorder, OCD, schizophrenia, etc). He absolutely states that brain disorders (including autism) are caused by mitochondria which are not working properly.[11] He emphasises the critical role of healthy mitochondria in both physical and mental health, including their involvement in gene expression, inflammation, and brain development.

This idea has a lot of scientific support. It also means we parents have more control. If we improve a child's mitochondrial health through improving their metabolic health, by changing what they eat, cleaning out toxins, giving them extra supplements, and by doing activities with them to grow their cerebellum, we can unlock their potential. This is what the 7-Step Autism Action Plan aims to do, and I will be guiding you step by step on how to do this for your child.

Mindset

The first step to learning any new skill or to making any progress at all in a new area is to believe that you, as a parent, can do this. With the right mindset and motivation, a person can achieve anything, beyond what they ever expected. This is essential for you as a parent to believe this, and to understand the expansive potential of the human brain and of neuroplasticity to change your child's inputs and therefore change their life outcomes.

To help address your mindset, a useful exercise to do would be to write down all your limiting beliefs that you have for yourself and for your child, and to ask yourself what the origin of that limiting belief is? Is this limiting belief even true/absolutely 100% true? Is the opposite of this limiting belief true? And then to write an affirmation which you should recite daily to create a new belief in your mind, overwriting that limiting belief.[12]

Scan the QR code on the next page to use the "Worksheet: Limiting Beliefs" to do this. The worksheet will help you discover:

- What is my limiting belief?
- Where did this belief come from?
- Is this limiting belief 100% true?
- Is this the opposite of this true?
- What is a positive affirmation I can use instead?

I have included a personal example in this worksheet too. When I first did this exercise I had over 40 limiting beliefs written down. The affirmation portion of the exercise is important, as a belief in the brain cannot be deleted. It needs to be overwritten with a new belief.

Once you have completed this exercise, start reciting your affirmations everyday (morning or evening is best) to make sure you are in the right mindset to believe you can help your child.

Before you start the 7-Step Autism Action Plan for your child, it is important to know what your developmental goals are for your child for the next 12 months. Writing down your goals and the reasons you have for these goals is always a helpful first step to know what direction you plan to go in as a parent and why. Use the "Worksheet: Goals and Motivation" on page 20 to help you do this.

In the next chapter, I will explain step 1, the power of oxytocin, and why it has to be the parent who helps unlock their autistic child's potential, and not external experts.

Key Takeaways:

- ❖ Neuroplasticity is the name given for the ability to create new brain connections and reorganise and prune your old brain connections. Understanding neuroplasticity means understanding there is the potential to change the brain you currently have or the brain you are born with.

- ❖ Early Years Intervention is important. There is a period of rapid growth in the brain from 0-5 years, which is when parents start seeing autism symptoms in their child. Intervening then means you have a greater influence in how your child's brain is wired, and how it grows.

- ❖ There is nothing wrong with the label "autism." But labels in general can be self-limiting or self-fulfilling. The symptoms of autism often come with a child experiencing a developmental delay, sensory overwhelm/underwhelm, or chronic anxiety/aggression, and these symptoms can predispose them to having other mental health conditions such as depression or bipolar disorder, etc.

- ❖ Epigenetics means genes can be switched on and off. Being born with a gene for autism does not necessarily mean autism symptoms have to be expressed, and this is shown for identical twins too.

❖ Beginning a lifestyle program to improve your child's metabolic health can improve their mitochondrial function, improve their physical health, and unlock their potential. Changing these environmental inputs for your child will rewire your child's brain through neuroplasticity, therefore leading to different behaviour expressions for your child.

Worksheet: How Do I Know If My Child Even Has Autism? (A Quiz)

Sometimes it can be difficult to know if your child is having typical autism symptoms or is just developing a bit slower than normal. Use this quiz below as a screening test to help you with this.

Usually children will need to have at least two of the following items in the list to be considered on the Autism Spectrum Disorder. The more symptoms that the child has from the list below, the greater chance that they have autism.

Answer each question with a "yes" or "no."

1. Social Communication Challenges:

- Does your child have difficulty understanding or using spoken language?

- Does your child struggle with understanding gestures, eye contact, or facial expressions?

- Does your child struggle with verbal and non-verbal communication?

- Does your child have a speech delay?

- Does your child have difficulty recognising emotions and intentions in others?

2. Restricted, Repetitive Behaviours:

- Does your child engage in repetitive stimming movements or have specific routines?

- Does your child have unusual obsessive interests?

3. Sensory Issues:

- Does your child show over- or under-sensitivities to sounds, lights, touch, tastes, smells, balance, or other stimuli?

4. Delayed Language, Motor, and Cognitive Skills:

- Does your child experience delays in language, motor, or cognitive skills?

5. Hyperactivity, Impulsivity, and/or Inattentive Behaviour:

- Does your child exhibit hyperactivity, impulsivity, and/or poor attention skills?

6. Gut Symptoms:

- Does your child commonly have loose stools, constipation, bloating, abdominal pain, gas or nausea symptoms?

7. Does your child show impulsive behaviour, with a limited sense of danger?

8. Does your child have unusual eating or sleeping habits?

9. Did your child experience a regression between the ages of 18 months to 3.5 years old, where they lost skills they previously had?

It's important to note that the way these symptoms manifest can vary widely among individuals with autism, and not all individuals will have the same set of symptoms or to the same degree.

Additionally, some symptoms may change over time or be influenced by the individual's environment and experiences.

Worksheet: Goals and Motivation

Write down 3-4 developmental goals that you have for yourself and your autistic child for the next 12 months.
1.

2.

3.

4.

List all of your reasons why you have these goals for yourself and your child. The more reasons you have for why you want to achieve these goals, the better.
1.

2.

3.

4.

5.

6.

7.

8.

9.

10.

11.

12.

13.

14.

15.

Part 1:
Core Concepts

Chapter 1
Step 1: Optimise Oxytocin

"Oxytocin is the great facilitator of life. It's an antidote to the fight-or-flight response."
- Daniel Goleman

In this chapter we are going to explore the significance of oxytocin, its impact on the brain and how we can hack this hormone to increase its levels in your autistic child.

Oxytocin is famously known as the "love hormone." Increasing oxytocin levels in your autistic child will help them to learn new skills faster, especially social skills. It will also help in the regulation of their emotional responses, pain perception, and for their hunger cues to become more consistent.

When oxytocin floods your brain, it helps regulate emotional responses and pro-social behaviours, such as trust, empathy, gazing, and positive memories. It also plays a role in enhancing sociality, affiliation, mind reading, and social memory.[13] These are all skills that symptomatic autistic children find difficult to learn. To help them learn these skills and behaviours (and other developmental skills), we need to flood their brain with oxytocin.

Oxytocin has an important role in facilitating learning for all humans. As well as learning, it helps regulate anxiety, feeding, and pain perception.[14] Again these are all things that your autistic child is struggling with. As a parent of an autistic child, my son was very anxious even in familiar spaces. He couldn't feel hunger, and sometimes went a few days only eating one bite of food, and he scarily never reacted to any pain. Where he hurt himself and a neurotypical child would have started crying and expressed pain, my son never reacted. It was eerie. Thankfully he doesn't do this anymore and now reacts normally to pain.

My client's autistic children can often be head bangers or self-harmers. As pain perception is regulated differently for autistic children, they often aren't even aware that they are hurting themselves and that they are supposed to be feeling pain. These are very scary events for all parents and onlookers. A boost in oxytocin could help them in regulating aggression, and promote social memory, attachment, bonding, and trust too.[15]

Knowing the importance of oxytocin for learning, aggression and anxiety regulation, and for building social skills, the next question is important: How can I flood my child's brain with oxytocin?

This is where you may be looking for a local pharmacy to try and buy some off-the-shelf oxytocin to inject into your child, and thus have a socially regulated child in all environments; and a child who has excellent pain and hunger perception and social skills. But if only life were that easy. Sadly there is a little bit more work than that. Oxytocin given intravenously struggles to cross the blood brain barrier.[16] Hence oxytocin needs to flood the brain naturally and it needs to be paired with behavioural therapy to enhance learning.[17]

What this means is that we need to promote natural oxytocin release in the child, and pair this with someone who they can bond/trust with to help them learn the skills they need that they may be developmentally delayed for. A natural person for this would be a child's parent or a child's teacher who they have a close 1:1 relationship with and see very often.

I've listed 6 methods below for you to try at home with your child to promote a natural oxytocin release in your child. For best results, combine the methods.

Boosting your child's oxytocin levels will enhance their learning, social skills, pain perception, hunger perception, emotional regulation, and decrease their anxiety levels—things that your autistic child may already be struggling with.

Method 1:
Spend at least 10-30 minutes a day 1:1 bonding time with your child, with all phones/screens put away, doing something that your child wants to do.

This seems simple, but I know it isn't. Often autistic children are in their own worlds, so to enter their world to bond with them isn't an easy task. Autistic children can often have unusual interests too. An example of how one of my clients did this, is that their 1.5-year-old son Thomas enjoyed watching lights spin around (visually stimming) for hours, and running up and down repetitively, not engaging with their surroundings. In order to bond with Thomas in a way that he was interested in, his parents sat with him on their lap or next to him uninterrupted everyday to watch those lights spin around and commenting on it at the same time. They also ran with Thomas up and down the hallways when he did this. Doing this activity or a similar activity with your autistic child for 10-30 minutes a day consistently will help compound results.

After a few weeks, Thomas began to notice his parents joining him on this. In his eyes, they had now entered his world and the parent-child bond deepened for him. Thomas began to communicate this to his parents by showing them more affection.

For your child it may be a few months and not a few weeks, but the key thing is being consistent. With consistency, the results will compound and like Thomas's, your child's brain will also get more and more flooded with oxytocin and they will learn social skills and all other skills faster.

As a disclaimer, I would like to say that as a busy working adult who is often a parent to other children too, finding 10-30 minutes a day to do what we would consider a "boring" activity is difficult. It's not easy to do this consistently. But to encourage you, remind yourself every day of your goals and your motivation: What is your *why* for committing to this? Knowing the answer to this will help you stay consistent. If you have completed the "Worksheet: Goals and Motivation", display this somewhere where you can see it every day. If you have someone to keep you accountable, e.g. a coach or a close group of friends, having that kind of support could also be really helpful.

Method 2:

Listen to music! Hearing and interacting with happy music, especially the act of singing in a group, has the ability to increase oxytocin levels.

Slow tempo and relaxing music, in particular, have been associated with increased salivary oxytocin levels. They also lower heart rates and stress levels in humans.[18]

One of the main characteristics of autistic children is often a speech delay and slower language and communication skills. You may be surprised to learn that the processing of music and language depends on the same brain system (the auditory and language centre), which is based in the temporal lobe of the brain. Functional imaging studies have revealed that some core elements of the brain's music and language systems are processed in closely related brain regions, but the wiring for these systems are different, and this causes the differences in functionality.

Music affects many aspects of human behaviour, especially in encouraging social interactions and promoting trust and cooperation within groups of people, something that symptomatic autistic individuals can struggle with. Music also impacts the limbic system in the brain, so listening to it is intrinsically rewarding and motivating, and music can facilitate aspects of learning and memory again through boosting oxytocin levels.

Knowing this, you can boost your autistic child's oxytocin levels through daily music. A classic way to do this is to sing nursery rhymes together (even when your child can't join in yet). Singing nursery rhymes has been proven to significantly contribute to a child's speech and language development.[19]

Nursery rhymes are repetitive, include actions, and teach rhythm and rhyme, which are all beneficial for speech, understanding, and language skills. They help children segment words into syllables, hear similarities between words that rhyme or start with the same sounds, and develop a sense of humour. Singing nursery rhymes also provides comfort and support to youngsters and introduces them to the idea of storytelling, promoting social skills and boosting language development as well as that all important love hormone oxytocin.[20]

Research has shown that infants learn languages from rhythmic information, such as the rise and fall of tone in nursery rhymes, and that speaking to babies using sing-song speech, like nursery rhymes, helps them learn language.[21]

My favourite nursery rhymes to sing to my children (especially between 0-5 years of age) were Row Row Your Boat, Wheels on the Bus, Wind the Bobbin Up, and Pat-A-Cake. These all have actions which you can do with your child. If you're unfamiliar with any of these nursery rhymes, you can find them all on YouTube too!

Lots of group singing is important as well. If you live close to a local library in the UK, it is likely they will host a nursery rhyme time a few times a week, which you can join in on. If your child is uncomfortable with loud sounds and musical instruments at the library rhyme time, then work your way up to this by just joining for the first 5 minutes and then eventually building your way up to the full 30-minute session.

Even if your child is uncomfortable with the first five minutes, stay with your child to comfort them through the experience, while allowing them to enjoy the cognitive and brain-boosting benefits of music.

Method 3:
Engage in high-intensity exercise.[22] This suggestion may not be a surprising one as there doesn't seem to be a problem that regular exercise can't help solve or prevent!

High-intensity exercise has been found to increase oxytocin levels in children, including those with autism. Additionally, studies have demonstrated that structured physical exercise, such as attending a martial arts or a gymnastics group class, can have a positive impact on socialisation and communication skills among children with autism, potentially due to its influence on oxytocin levels.[23] While the exact mechanisms behind the relationship between high-intensity exercise and how it works to boost oxytocin levels in autistic children are still being explored, the evidence suggests that engaging in such structured physical high-intensity exercise activities may help boost oxytocin production, which could in turn positively impact social behaviours and well-being for autistic children.

Knowing this, I enrolled my son into a group gymnastics class and a group martial arts class from the age of three. Getting there on time each week with my son and a newborn was tough, and then watching the lessons from the window in the door was even harder. My son had a gross motor delay and he didn't really listen to instructions well, and he was sort of in his own world. I used to always find myself mentally comparing him to the other children his age, who used to have much more sophisticated physical skills and had much better attention skills than my son.

After he attended the martial arts lessons consistently for one year, the teacher said to me, "I don't think he's ready to attend, he is too young, and you might be better off stopping the lessons and returning when he's started school."

I didn't listen to her. I replied "I still want him to attend, I think he'll be learning more being here with the other children in this environment than he would at home." So we carried on. And four months later, like a light switch, the teacher saw some progress and told me he was ready to grade for his first belt.

As you can imagine, I was over the moon! I knew there would eventually be progress, but I also managed my expectations that all progress he would make would be slow. By this time, the children he had started with were already grading for their third belts, but my son was only just starting to grade for his first belt. It is hard as a parent to stop the mental comparisons, but I always tried to remind myself to compare his progress with how he was 6 months ago, or 12 months ago, not to the other children of similar ages around him.

Method 4:
Utilise the simple act of touch to boost oxytocin release. Giving someone a massage, cuddling, or hugging leads

to higher levels of this hormone and a greater sense of well-being.[24]

I am someone who came from a home where we didn't really show any physical affection, so this is a new behaviour that I really had to learn.

For children with autism, there are often two different responses to physical touch. Some kids with autism might feel things more intensely when they are touched, and certain textures or sensations might be overwhelming for them or bother them.

Whereas some children with autism may seek out or enjoy physical touch, others may only find it comfortable in specific contexts or forms.[25] The experiences and responses to physical touch can vary widely among children with autism, so it is important to understand where your child is in this spectrum.

If your child seeks out physical touch, then lean into this as much as you can, and be generous with your hugs, cuddles, and hand holding. If your child is aversive to physical touch, then try including this behaviour slowly, gently stroking your child and slowly increasing the length of time you can do this. If you stick to this program for 12-16 months, your child's autism symptoms should reduce, and progress should be made towards their developmental milestones, helping to unlock their potential. Hence at the end of these 12 months, your child may surprise you and begin to seek out physical touch and affection from you, or show you that they are enjoying this more when you hug or touch them.

Method 5:

Get used to laughing together, as laughter leads to the release of oxytocin and endorphins. This might be a feeling you've already experienced, when you are laughing at the same time as someone else and you both look at each other, you will feel more bonded to that person in that moment. This is due to the release of oxytocin and endorphins occurring in those moments, which encourages people to connect and have friendly interactions with each other.

As a parent, try and maybe watch a child-friendly comedy movie or puppet show together as a way to bond with your autistic child. Doing so may trigger the release of oxytocin in the child, therefore improving their learning skills.

I know how boring some of these children's shows are. But if you can spend time with your child, and even fake laugh while gazing in your child's eyes as they are laughing, you may notice the social bonding and oxytocin levels increase between you both.

Method 6:

Consider caring for a pet dog or a pet cat (if you don't have one yet). This is my favourite method for autistic families and works particularly amazingly well if your autistic child has aggressive tendencies or frequent emotional meltdowns.

The benefits of having a pet dog (or a pet cat) as a companion pet for an autistic family is numerous. Dogs have a very sophisticated sense of smell and can detect all sorts of emotions a child and adult are feeling through their sense of smell. An intelligent calm temperament companion dog, such as a golden retriever, a labrador or a labradoodle, can be a wonderful calming influence for someone who has autism. An affectionate dog provides unconditional love and friendship on a daily basis. There have been a multitude of studies which show that interaction between dog owners and their dogs results in increasing levels of oxytocin in both owners and dogs.[26] Which means when pet owners say that their dog loves them, this can be scientifically proven too!

Walking the dog provides both fresh air and exercise for your autistic child, and can also have the unexpected benefit of easing social situations with other children too. Learning to care for the dog teaches responsibility and practical skills. And pets provide parents with opportunities to teach and model caring behaviours and consideration of a friend's needs—both important social skills which all children, especially autistic children, may struggle to learn.

It is possible to find a service dog or a therapy dog which could help navigate an autistic child through their environment and help to calm a child down. They can also help stop self-injurious behaviours, which some autistic children can frequently engage in. Dogs are gifted with more emotional intelligence than most humans, and trained therapy or service dogs learn when to go for a hug or when to lean back with their autistic child.

There is also a sensory stimulation benefit which autistic children can benefit from when stroking their pet's fur. Some of my clients' families who have purchased a service dog or a therapy dog for their autistic child often rave about how it really calms their autistic child down, and thus calms the family home down.

The choice to purchase a companion dog, service dog, or a therapy dog does depend on the resources and commitment of the family. However, as a precaution, it is important to test if the autistic child (or anyone else living in the family home) has a sensitivity or allergy to dogs or cats by doing a skin test before purchasing a pet.

There are also some breeds which can equally be well trained, e.g. a cavapoo which can be more allergy friendly. So testing any allergy responses to a more allergy-friendly breed can be a consideration if someone living in the family home does have a sensitivity to pets.

Key Takeaways:

- ❖ Oxytocin is often called the love hormone. It helps regulate emotions like trust and empathy. Autistic children often struggle with these skills, so boosting oxytocin will help them learn better.

- ❖ Oxytocin not only aids in learning but also helps with anxiety, hunger perception, and pain sensitivity. Autistic children may have difficulties in these areas, so increasing oxytocin levels will be beneficial.

- ❖ You can naturally increase oxytocin levels in your child through activities like bonding time, listening to music, high-intensity exercise, physical touch, laughter and having a pet dog or cat.

- ❖ Using a combination of these methods can be most effective in boosting oxytocin levels and helping your autistic child learn new skills and regulate their emotions better.

- ❖ By increasing oxytocin levels in your child, you can promote neuroplasticity and help rewire their brain, leading to improved social skills and emotional regulation. Using a variety of methods can provide the best chance of success.

Chapter 2
Step 2: Break Down Blood

"When it comes to diagnosis, a blood test is often the first step in ruling out other medical conditions and ensuring an accurate assessment." - Unknown

Often there are reasons other than Autism to explain a child's symptoms, such as a vitamin or mineral deficiency, or an autoimmune disorder. It is important to exclude these factors in determining if there are any other explanations for your child's symptoms. The best way to do this is to approach your GP asking for a blood test for your child to test for specific biomarkers. If the blood test shows your child lacks certain things or has an unusual profile, your GP can help fix that to make them healthier.

Not performing this step poses a risk of overlooking underlying medical reasons for your child's behaviour.

For instance, if your child has low iron levels, which is only truly diagnosable through a blood test, this may go undetected by the parent or their GP. Correcting an iron deficiency is crucial as iron levels impact neurotransmitter production, including dopamine and serotonin, which are vital for mood regulation. Therefore, ensuring your child undergoes a blood test is essential for their physical wellbeing and emotional regulation. I have listed the reasons for why each biomarker should be tested for in their blood test below.

The blood tests that you should ask your GP to test for should include the following:

Serum Iron Levels

Serum iron levels directly measure the iron in the blood. Optimal iron levels are crucial for brain development as iron plays a key role in producing neurotransmitters, impacting brain function and mood regulation.[27] Adequate iron levels are essential for optimal brain development, crucial for your child to learn new skills. Iron also supports energy production, immune function, and physical growth.

Ferritin

Ferritin measures the body's iron stores and contributes to dopamine production in the body.[28] Dopamine is a crucial neurotransmitter which regulates sleep, focus, and concentration.[29] These are areas often challenging for autistic children. If a child's ferritin levels are low, this would exacerbate any sleep, focus, and concentration problems that the child may already have. Correcting a body's low ferritin level with a supplement prescription is simple for GPs to do.

Complete Blood Count (CBC)

A complete blood count will measure Haemoglobin, Haematocrit, Red Blood Cell levels, and Platelet levels in the child. If a blood test shows an abnormality in Haemoglobin, Haematocrit or Red Blood Cell levels, this can be associated with having nutritional deficiencies, such as iron deficiency anaemia or vitamin deficiencies.[30] A CBC is essential to learn a child's nutritional status and whether they are absorbing their food correctly.

White Blood Cells (WBC) Count

If a child has an abnormality in their WBC count, it might show as an infection or an immune system issue. If a child's WBC is abnormal, the underlying causes must also be investigated and determined by the GP.

C-Reactive Protein

This is an inflammatory marker. If it is high, it could indicate chronic inflammation occurring. Or it could be a sign of the child having an autoimmune disorder.

Examples of possible autoimmune conditions include: ulcerative colitis or a leaky gut, which is particularly common in autistic children.[31] If a child's C-Reactive protein is high, the underlying causes must be investigated and determined by the GP.

Thyroid Panel (TSH, T4, T3 and Iodine Levels)

If a child's thyroid hormones are all high, the child can have trouble sleeping, irritability, be hot all the time, or be anxious.[32] If their thyroid hormones are all low then the child can be depressed, more constipated, their skin could be dry, their hair brittle, and they often can't think clearly.[33] Similarly, these are symptoms that autistic children can likely present with and they can easily be corrected by the GP with the appropriate prescription.

Complete Metabolic Profile

Ordering this blood test will test a child's blood sugar levels, kidney and liver functioning. Testing the function of these organs are important as they provide an insight to how well your child's body is detoxifying.

Total Cholesterol Levels

Low levels of cholesterol are associated with depression and death from all causes for children and for adults.[34] Hence a child's cholesterol level should be within the optimum range and children should be encouraged to eat a high unsaturated fat diet, i.e. avocados, extra virgin olive oil, salmon, nuts and seeds. Children should also avoid eating products advertised as being low in fat or "0% fat" as this is linked to depression and can encourage overeating.

Total Carnitine

This includes testing for Free Carnitine and Acylcarnitines. These biomarkers are vital to helping develop a child's language acquisition and their muscle tone,[35] something autistic children can typically struggle with. Therefore carnitine levels should also be optimised within an autistic child.

Vitamin D

This is the feel-good hormone. Having low Vitamin D levels is associated with Autism, ADHD, Cancer and Depression.[36] If a blood test shows that your child is low in Vitamin D, this can also be easily optimised within your child through vitamin D supplementation by your child's GP.

Vitamin B12

Having low levels of Vitamin B12 is linked to having anxiety and poor overall health.[37] Adequate Vitamin B12 levels are essential for children's growth, development and cognitive development. Therefore it is essential for your child's GP to test for this to promote a child's overall health and development. As autistic children can often have a history of fussy eating, there is a greater risk of lower vitamin levels compared to neurotypical children.

Omega 3 Index

This is tested through a finger prick test. Usually GPs do not test for Omega 3 levels, so this is something that parents can arrange themselves through finding an online provider to order an at-home test kit. It is important to measure a child's Omega 3 levels as autistic kids can typically have a 1% or lower Omega-3 index, whereas children with ADD/ADHD kids can often have an Omega 3 index of 3% or lower.[38] An optimum level is between 8%-12% and this can easily be achieved through making dietary changes for the child or using supplementation. Omega 3 is very important for improving cognitive function, focus and for reducing inflammation levels in the body.[39] Hence it is very important to measure a child's Omega 3 index to understand what their baseline level is.

Lyme Disease

If your child has ever had a history of a tick bite, you should ask your doctor to perform this test. The symptoms of lyme disease can have a crossover with some of the symptoms of autism. For example lyme disease can also cause fatigue and sensory processing issues.[40] Lyme disease is also easily treatable so it is important to rule it out as a cause of your child's symptoms.

Next Steps

Please scan the QR code below to download a table detailing biomarker level ranges for a healthy child and optimal level ranges for a child. This will allow you to identify any deviations from optimal functioning and take corrective actions through supplementation or prescription if necessary to help your child.

The table does differentiate between what an optimum level is for a child, and what is the normal reference level for a child, as sometimes a biomarker level can be considered normal, but not optimal. For example, in the case of the Omega-3 Index, research suggests that an optimal range for general wellness and health outcomes is between 8-12%. This range is associated with better health outcomes for the heart, brain, eyes, and joints.[41]

While most people globally have an Omega-3 Index below 8%, aiming for a higher range within 8-12% is linked to improved health. Using a narrower optimal range to assess a blood test result can help you as a parent to detect any imbalances early on, and address them proactively to optimise your child's health rather than just detect clinical abnormalities.

Once you have your child's test results, work with your GP to improve your child's health. If there are deficiencies, you can work on them to enhance your child's physical health and emotional well-being. Often for my clients, these tests will show a deficiency in at least one or more areas.

For my own son, I had to fight the GP for a blood test, as they don't often perform blood tests for children aged two without an obvious medical need. I saw on the letter from the GP explaining the results that it included the note "Mum insisted for a blood test." And I am so happy that I did insist on doing the blood test, as since then my son has had a prescription for Ferritin. My son's omega-3 index was also very low.

It is sad that as parents of autistic children we need to navigate the system in a certain way in order to secure the appropriate help and support for our children. As parents, we have the right to advocate for our children's needs and request necessary tests to identify any potential concerns. Your child's GP should be acting as your partner, and we have a right to request a blood test for our children to identify any outliers.

Key Takeaways:

- ❖ Sometimes symptoms in children might not only be due to autism, but could be caused by other factors like vitamin deficiencies or autoimmune disorders. It's essential to rule out these possibilities to understand your child's health better.

- ❖ Asking your GP for a blood test is the best way to investigate potential underlying causes of your child's symptoms. This test can check various markers to see if your child lacks certain nutrients or has unusual profiles that need medical attention.

- ❖ If the blood test shows any deficiencies or abnormalities, it's an opportunity to work with your GP to address them. By fixing these issues, you can improve your child's overall health, helping them stay well and enhancing their ability to learn and develop new skills.

- ❖ Advocate for your child. Sometimes, getting the necessary medical tests for your child might require persistence and advocacy. As a parent, it's important to stand up for your child's needs and ensure they receive the appropriate care and support.

- ❖ By following these steps and collaborating with healthcare professionals, you can better understand and address any underlying health issues your child may have, ultimately supporting their overall well-being and development.

Part 2:
Cultivate & Cleanse

Chapter 3
Step 3: Grasp the Gut-Brain Bond

"The gut is like a second brain, influencing not only digestion but also mood, immune function, and cognitive abilities." - Dr Tim Spector

If you are unfamiliar with what is meant by "Gut Health", you may be rightly confused, thinking that the function of your gut is to be the organ which digests your food and makes your poop!

In reality, much of your mental health can be attributed to your gut function. There are more than 100 million brain cells in the gut which tells you that it's very powerful in thinking for itself.[42] Your gut also has more neurons (brain cells) than the spinal cord and the peripheral nervous system.[43]

The Gut Microbiome houses a vast array of microbial cells (10-100 Trillion to be precise!), within the gastrointestinal tract. These microbial cells include: bacteria, fungi, viruses, and other organisms.[44] This diverse community plays a pivotal role in maintaining both a person's physical and mental health. A healthy gut microbiome is a diverse gut microbiome where everything is in balance.[45] These gut microorganisms contribute to vital bodily functions including: digestion, immunity, protecting the gut lining and sending instructions to and from the brain via the gut-brain axis.[46]

Within the gut microbiome, there is a specific large and powerful community of microorganisms called the psychobiome, which directly influences a person's mood, mental health and behaviours.[47] The psychobiome has an intricate relationship with the nervous system that can be affected by diet, lifestyle, and environmental factors. Influencing the makeup of your child's psychobiome offers a crucial avenue for managing anxiety and stress in autistic children. Understanding all of these dynamics explains why the gut is nicknamed a person's "second brain."

Gut Health and Autism

Several studies, including from Harvard Medical School and Massachusetts Institute of Technology,[48] have found distinctive gut microbiome patterns in children with autism.[49] Children with autism often have changes in their gut, including increased wall permeability, higher levels of certain substances called endotoxins (markers showing stress from oxidation), and the presence of inflammatory cells. Crucially, how severe these levels and biomarkers are correlate with the severity of their autistic behavioural symptoms, emphasising the intricate connection between gut health and brain health.

An increase in gut wall permeability is most commonly called "Leaky Gut" syndrome, and it is very common in autistic children. Leaky gut syndrome is a condition in which tiny holes develop in the lining of the intestinal tract, letting things like bacteria and undigested food get into your bloodstream. This leads to chronic inflammation in the body and changes in your gut, which will affect a person's overall health.

Leaky gut syndrome has been associated with: autism, autoimmune disorders, digestive spectrum disorders, IBS, Crohn's disease, celiac disease, asthma, allergies, hormonal problems, depression, fibromyalgia, chronic fatigue syndrome, ADD, acne, rosacea, candida, food allergies and headaches.[50]

Understanding the significant role of the gut microbiome helps us to understand how having a leaky gut can affect so many different systems of the body, and that having a Leaky Gut is more common in children with autism symptoms. Almost half of children with autism suffer from at least one gastrointestinal symptom,[51] and they tend to suffer more from gastrointestinal symptoms as compared to neurotypical children,[52] with diarrhoea and constipation being the most common symptoms reported.[53]

In a healthy individual, food particles are absorbed in their small intestine. In Leaky Gut syndrome, a person's gut lining becomes more permeable, allowing food particles to enter the bloodstream before they are fully broken down in the small intestine. When these not-fully-broken-down food particles are absorbed into the bloodstream early, a person can become sensitised to it. The human immune system doesn't like anything foreign in the bloodstream so even if it's a piece of banana or rice, the immune system will create antibodies toward that banana/rice, and antibodies will then be fixed onto the small piece of banana, causing an inflammatory reaction in the person.

The brain will see that there is an inflammatory reaction occurring and will then, through a protective mechanism, influence your child's behaviour to become really dull and irritable, and they may start stimming. Healing a child's leaky gut means that child's behaviour will then improve, helping to unlock their potential.

Antibiotics treatment can also have a significant effect on gut health. Antibiotics treatment is similar to exploding a nuclear bomb on a child's gut health. It will not only kill any "bad bacteria" which is causing the infection, but it will kill the good bacteria in a child's gut too. Antibiotics use will significantly reduce gut bacteria diversity, affect digestion, and will disrupt the gut-brain connection.[54] Antibiotics use has been rising globally[55] and autistic children can often have a history of antibiotics consumption too.

The total and variety of gut bacteria in the gut decreases immediately after taking antibiotics, and it can take months and usually years for the gut microbiome to recover from a single course of antibiotics.[56] As parents of autistic children this can be worrying, as our children will be more vulnerable to having autism symptoms; therefore we should be more mindful about giving antibiotics. Of course if there is a life-and-death reason why a child should have a course of antibiotics, it is important to give the antibiotics! But while having the antibiotics and directly after, a program to heal the gut should begin immediately too.

Another way that an autistic child can have an unhealthy gut is if there is a yeast or bacterial overgrowth in their gut microbiome. These can cause a variety of symptoms in autistic children, including making it harder for them to be potty-trained or to remain dry overnight. An overgrowth of yeast in the gut can happen when there is too much cortisol (the body's stress hormone) in the body.[57] It is common for autistic children to have a higher level of cortisol in their bodies, as they are often stressed and their default is to be in the fight-flight-freeze mode. Just living in our world where they are experiencing a sensory overwhelm or underwhelm everyday can cause them a lot of daily stress.

Common Causes of Leaky Gut Syndrome

There are many causes of Leaky Gut syndrome which include: a high sugar or ultra high processed food diet, low stomach acid, alcohol or smoking, poor sleep, antibiotics use, artificial sweeteners, environmental toxins, stress, and a low fibre diet.[58]

A high-sugar diet can lead to changes in the gut microbiome, favouring the growth of unhealthy bacteria and yeasts, while suppressing the growth of beneficial bacteria. This imbalance in the makeup of the gut microbiome can lead to inflammation and damage to the gut lining, resulting in small holes appearing in the gut lining.[59]

Eating ultra-high processed foods can also cause a similar effect in a child's gut lining.

King's College London University professor, Dr Tim Spector, defined ultra-high processed foods as "edible food-like substances" that are created by taking the ingredients from real food, stripping away key components such as fibre, and adding various chemicals and additives to imitate the appearance of real food and increase their shelf life.[60] These foods typically have extensive packaging and may feature health claims, such as being high in protein, low in fats, or having no added sugar. Examples of ultra-high processed food include all supermarket bread, crisps, flavoured yoghurts, cereals, fizzy drinks, orange juice and other heavily processed items.

I like to think of ultra-high processed foods as any food that is either made in a factory, e.g. supermarket bread. Or if it is something that your great grandmother would not recognise as food or as a food ingredient, e.g. a fast food burger, fizzy drink or "emulsifier", then this should be classified as an ultra-high processed food. In the UK and in many other developed countries, more than half of their population's diets consist of eating ultra-high processed food which is a concerning modern trend.

If a child's stomach lining is inflamed, this can lead to a reduction in the production of their stomach acid, which can also contribute to leaky gut syndrome.[61] If a child is taking medication like omeprazole or lansoprazole (which is a Proton pump inhibitor) used to treat acid reflux in children over the age of one year old, this can contribute to a decrease in the production of their stomach acid.[62] Research has found that individuals with autism are more likely to have reflux or bloating issues as an infant/child, compared to those without autism, and so are more likely to have been prescribed this medication.[63]

Alcohol use can also cause a decrease in stomach acid production, but this shouldn't be relevant to autistic children except perhaps for children who also suffered from Foetal Alcohol Syndrome while in the womb. A systematic review and meta-analysis conducted by the University of Pisa reported that autism spectrum disorder is present at a rate almost two times higher in children with foetal alcohol syndrome.[64]

How to Improve Gut Health in Autistic Children
By now we understand the importance of the Gut-Brain connection and how poor gut health increases risk of

autism symptoms in children. There are many ways to improve the diversity of your child's gut microbiome and begin to heal their gut. The first way is to change their diet to become gluten-free and casein-free.

Gluten-Free and Casein-Free Diet

Changing to a Gluten-Free and Casein-Free diet for autistic children can be very effective at reducing or eliminating autism symptoms in autistic children.[65] Often, once gluten and casein have been eliminated from an autistic child's diet, a non-verbal autistic child may start to speak words within 6 weeks to 3 months of this change.

Autistic children will often have sensitivities to the Gluten protein and to the Casein protein (found within unfermented dairy products).[66] Eating gluten can trigger the release of a protein called zonulin, which can lead to increased gut wall permeability.[67] Zonulin is a protein that regulates the tight junctions of the gut, and when it is released, the tight junctions open slightly, causing holes in the gut wall and allowing larger particles to pass through. Research has identified small intestinal exposure to gluten as powerful triggers for zonulin to be released.

Eating gluten can sometimes cause a rare condition called Gluten Ataxia.[68] This condition happens when gluten makes the body's immune system react and harm the cerebellum part of the brain. This can lead to problems like clumsy movements, poor balance, and difficulty talking,[69] which are also common in autistic children. Treating gluten ataxia involves following a strict diet without gluten, which can help improve symptoms and stop more damage to the nervous system. Although gluten ataxia is not common, it shows that eating gluten can directly affect the brain and nervous system, and causes symptoms similar to those seen in autistic children. Gluten ataxia can occur in individuals with or without Coeliac's Disease.

There is an area of the brain called the hippocampus, whose primary function is making new memories. Gluten has been associated with decreasing the size of the hippocampus,[70] which makes learning new skills harder. Gluten is also an addictive substance and has proven opioid effects on the brain.[71] Hence once gluten is completely eliminated from a child's diet, withdrawal symptoms should be expected and will last no longer than 3 days. There are no nutritional benefits exclusive to gluten that cannot be found from other dietary sources. Therefore, it is entirely possible to maintain a balanced and healthy diet without eating gluten.

Autistic children often have an intolerance to casein, especially alpha and beta casein found in unfermented dairy products, like cow's milk. Gamma casein, found in fermented dairy, like kefir, is generally better tolerated.

During the human digestion process, alpha and βeta casein found in unfermented dairy products such as cow's milk, can mix with stomach acid and turn into a morphine-like peptide substance.[72] This can also bind to the opioid centres of the brain and can cause an addiction. In addition, 65% of the global population do not have an enzyme to digest lactose in milk,[73] which makes the digestion of this protein difficult. Gluten and Alpha/βeta casein can also commonly cause diarrhoea, colicky pain in children, and constipation (leading to a disruptive expansive gut pain for autistic children)—all of which can wake a child up at night.[74]

Gluten and αlpha/β-casein can both cause a functional folate deficiency in children, as they both block the folate receptors in the brain.[75] As most children with autism are already low in folate in their brains, so eating gluten and unfermented dairy products (which will have large amounts of αlpha/β-casein in them) can make that problem worse. Folate is critical for proper brain function. Cerebral folate deficiency has been shown to be a problem in many children with autism.[76]

Therefore in this process, unfermented dairy products are first eliminated alongside gluten, and then the parent should see if there has been a behaviour change within their child. If after 6 weeks of completely making this change, an improvement in your child's symptoms has not been seen yet, only then should fermented dairy products also be eliminated.

All meal ideas featured in this book are gluten-free and casein-free for simplicity.

While modern society often associates ingesting medications with chemical reactions occurring in our bodies that can alleviate symptoms and cause unwanted side effects, the impact of food on our bodies is frequently neglected.

Eating different foods can trigger reactions leading to various symptoms, such as constipation, depression, anxiety, leaky gut, or behaviours linked to autism. Despite the average child eating significantly more food than they do medication annually, little consideration is given to the chemical and biological effects of their daily meals and snacks.

Prioritising dietary changes is typically the quickest route to improved health and well-being. This is true for both neurotypical individuals and for autistic children.

Recognising how important a healthy gut is for the brain shows that changing what we eat can really help alleviate autism symptoms.

To make this change in an autistic-child-friendly way is challenging, and it is best to do this gradually. For example, for my clients whose autistic children drink a lot of unfermented cow's milk in a bottle everyday, I would ask the parent to gradually reduce the amount of cow's milk in a bottle, and replace this with a dairy-free milk alternative.

Usually once this change has happened completely, within 2 months, a child will drink a whole bottle of dairy-free milk instead of cow's milk like they did previously. Another practical strategy is to first use the sweetened version of the dairy-free milk; this sweetened version of the milk can help your child adjust to the change.

A similar recommendation can be made for a gluten-free transition. Look at the meals your child is currently eating, and see if any substitutions can be made with gluten-free ingredients. Gradually change the pasta or bread your child eats to become gluten-free. Have an aim that within three months, all of their meals will become wholly gluten free.

Another great substitute to make is to use grass-fed, organic ghee instead of butter/margarine when cooking your child's meals. Grass-fed organic ghee is casein free (and lactose free!). You can use "Worksheet: Meal Ideas" to help you make this change.

As a parent, you will know your child's situation best. However a gradual transition to alpha/beta casein-free and gluten-free meals and drinks is usually the most realistic method to achieve this transition, while the parents and child both adjust to this change.

Sometimes if a child's bowels do not approve after removing gluten and casein from their diet, it can be indicative of having a yeast or bacterial infection. So it would then be recommended to decompress the gut to alleviate the constipation with a high-fibre diet and high-fibre supplement, which I will talk about next.

Increasing Dietary Fibre

Eating more fibre helps keep our child's gut healthy by feeding the good bacteria. It also keeps their stomach working well and maintains the diversity of their gut microbiome. Examples of great fibre sources which can be added to your autistic child's diet to improve their gut health include: whole grain sourdough bread, steel cut porridge oats, brown rice, whole grain pasta, quinoa, apples (with the skin), bananas (particularly green bananas), strawberries, blueberries, carrots, and sweet potatoes.

I wanted to caveat that although sourdough bread technically does contain gluten, because of the 12-hour fermentation process that freshly baked sourdough bread must go through, this fermentation process breaks down the gluten in the bread. Hence in the majority of cases it can be considered a safe food for most autistic children to eat. In addition, sourdough bread is rich in nutrients, such as folate, magnesium, and potassium, and it is a prebiotic (so promotes the growth of beneficial gut bacteria).

As parents of autistic children, we know they can often be fussy eaters, so there are several tricks that I will share on how to get your children to eat these foods to try:

1. Puree fruit or vegetables and mix a safe amount discreetly into the foods they already eat. In my children's foods, I often discreetly puree up a small amount of fruit or vegetable of my choice into the sauce of their food when preparing it, so that they don't notice it or see the food. It is very important to start off small, perhaps one teaspoon of pureed fruit/vegetables to their safe food, and over time (maybe each week at a time), you can gradually increase this.

2. Fibre-rich snacks such as whole-grain crackers or bread sticks can be great. These beige snacks can be quite bland-tasting, so are suitable for autistic children. If you are buying these from the supermarket, make sure they don't have any extra preservatives or other ingredients in them that you wouldn't find in a typical kitchen cupboard.

3. Beans/Legumes in burgers or meatballs. Adding finely mashed black beans or lentils to burgers or meatballs can be a great tip. The taste and texture are often disguised to the child by the other ingredients.

4. Fruit and Veggie ice lollies. It is usually quick and easy to make ice lollies in your freezer using blended fruits and vegetables. The cold sensation can distract from the texture, and the sweetness of the fruits can mask the veggie taste.

5. Mix chia seeds into full fat yoghurt. Many of my clients will eat yoghurts, and mixing chia seeds into a full fat dairy-free yoghurt or a pudding means that the seeds will absorb the liquid and develop a gel-like consistency. This adds fibre into your child's diet without altering the taste much. It is possible that your child will not like

seeing the black dots of the chia seeds in their food, so begin with a small portion, or distract them while they are eating so that they don't notice the black dots.

6. A very popular technique for my own children and for many of my clients is to add a tasteless odourless and kid-friendly soluble fibre supplement to the food that they are already eating. They will be eating this extra fibre source everyday without even noticing!

I also won't pretend these are all easy steps to take. I would say the weaning process for my son took at least 3.5 to 4 years, not the 6 months that mums are promised by health visitors! And it was difficult! My son didn't feel hunger, was an extremely fussy eater and his weight moved up and down the weight percentiles frequently.

It was constantly tough, and it required a great deal of perseverance and consistency from me. After what seemed like a very long time, his habits did change. The more you heal your child's gut, the less they will show the autistic symptoms of sensory overload from the textures and tastes. And slowly, slowly, they also become better eaters. The earlier you heal your child's gut, the easier it will be for them to adapt to these dietary changes long term.

As busy working parents, I would recommend to meal prep your children's foods as much as possible, and to utilise your slow cooker and freezer! This is one of the best ways to have healthy food available to eat at mealtimes without the rush. The best fibre-rich dishes to meal-prep for your children are Sweet Potato and Black Bean Tortilla Wraps, Baked Chicken Tenders with Sweet Potato Fries, and Banana-Oat Muffins.

<u>Use Prebiotics and Probiotics</u>

A common question I hear is what is the difference between prebiotics and probiotics? Prebiotics are a food source for the good gut bacteria in your gut, whereas Probiotics are a type of food which contain the beneficial bacteria themselves.

Prebiotics help make the good bacteria grow in the child's large intestine, and therefore improve their gut health. Probiotics work to repair the gut wall to make this less leaky and decrease any gut inflammation occurring.

Examples of Prebiotics and Probiotics food which are autistic child-friendly include:
- Bananas which can be served as a snack by itself or mashed up into other foods
- Sliced apples (with or without the skin)
- Strawberries or Blueberries

- Homemade Hummus made from Chickpeas
- Sweet Potatoes (baked or mashed)
- Carrot sticks
- Coconut Yoghurt or Almond Yoghurt
- Quinoa
- Brown Rice
- Chia seeds mixed into yoghurts or smoothies (even a small amount is great)
- Chia seed pudding (using dairy free milk)
- Ground flax seeds sprinkled on porridge or yoghurt
- Dairy Free cheese

As some of these prebiotics and probiotics can have a distinct taste if your child isn't used to it, only use very small amounts (even just 1 teaspoon) at meal times to begin with. Even 1 teaspoon consistently is small enough to make a difference to your child's gut microbiome, as 1 teaspoon will contain tens of millions of prebiotic bacteria in it.

Elimination Diet
For children with severe autistic symptoms persisting after 3-6 months of implementing these dietary changes, or those with atypical symptoms like hallucinations or brain fog, an Elimination Diet might be worth trying for three weeks. During this period, eliminate sugar, gluten, dairy, maize, soy, eggs, nuts, prawns, artificial dyes and

sweeteners from the diet. After three to four weeks, reintroduce one food type at a time, noting any changes in behaviour or symptoms. This helps identify any foods exacerbating autism symptoms, which can then be avoided. Keeping a daily diary can help correlate changes in behaviour with diet and reinforce positive effects of dietary changes for parents.

It's best to try these dietary changes under supervision of a qualified dietician. However, NHS dietician appointments in the UK often have long waits, risking your child missing crucial early years intervention time. This is why I wrote this book and created my program—to ensure parents like me have access to this information and can learn to help themselves to support their child during this critical time.

Organic, Free-Range Meat without Pesticides

Consider the state of farming in the UK, where many farms practise "zero-grazing," confining animals indoors without access to sunlight or fields. These animals often endure distress and depression, producing chemicals associated with depression. Eating the animal products from these farms may expose us to these chemicals, potentially contributing to rising rates of depression and mental health issues in society.

Additionally, many crops in the UK are sprayed with pesticides, which can negatively impact gut health with continuous exposure. To mitigate this, opt for organic fruits, vegetables, eggs, and meat whenever possible. However, in the UK even organic labelling doesn't guarantee freedom from pesticides, though levels are typically lower.

If organic options are unavailable, consider peeling fruits and vegetables and washing them thoroughly with sodium bicarbonate to minimise pesticide residue. While peeling may not eliminate all pesticides, it reduces overall exposure, lessening disruption to your child's gut microbiome. During periods of rapid brain growth, like pregnancy or early childhood, prioritise purchasing only organic foods if possible.

Thirty Plants A Week
According to Professor Tim Spector of King's College London University, a person should aim to eat at least thirty plants a week. This can sound daunting at first. However, when you realise that Spector classifies anything that comes from the ground as a plant—including herbs, spices, nuts, seeds in even small doses—towards eating the thirty plants a week, this can be achievable as long as you are cooking the meals at home yourself. By cooking meals at home, especially non-western dishes like Pakistani curries, which are rich

in spices, herbs and seeds, reaching thirty plants a week becomes achievable. If your child has an ethnic cuisine, then eating similar foods to how their ethnic ancestors ate is important for promoting a healthy and diverse gut microbiome.[77]

During my son's severe autism symptoms, he had no appetite and was underweight. I focused on ensuring that even one bite of food he consumed was a plant-filled Pakistani curry with organic ingredients. For the health of his gut microbiome, small amounts of these foods regularly will compound to have a positive impact over time.

To promote your child's brain health, eat wild-caught baked fish weekly and prioritise foods rich in healthy fats, like wild salmon, avocado, nuts, eggs, and dairy-free dark chocolate (70% or more). Avoid low-fat diets and opt for cooking oils such as avocado oil, extra virgin olive oil or organic ghee, while steering clear of omega-6-rich vegetable oils. Additionally, limit refined sugar intake and use alternative sweeteners like stevia or erythritol sparingly.

Gut Testing

If you've made these lifestyle changes consistently for your child without seeing improvements in their symptoms or behaviour after three months, consider seeking testing for their gut health. Look for a provider offering a 3-day stool test, Organic Acids Test (OATS) of their urine, and a blood sugar test. These tests can identify parasites, yeast infections, and nutritional deficiencies affecting metabolic pathways. The Gut Intuition, a London-based company, can offer this testing. Securing these tests for your autistic child through an overstretched NHS will be challenging.

Mindset

Making these lifestyle and dietary changes may be challenging for your family, requiring adjustments like reading food labels, shopping for different groceries, and cooking more at home. To help you through this transition, consider the following tips:

1. Write down your reasons for making these changes and display them where you can see them daily (use "Worksheet: Goals and Motivation" to help you to do this!)
2. Plan your meals and grocery lists in advance to make healthier food decisions.
3. Keep track of your child's diet and symptoms daily in a journal to monitor progress.

Maintaining a positive mindset is crucial. As your child's gut heals and their gut-brain connection strengthens, you may notice improvements in speech, eye contact, and sleep within three to four weeks.

To avoid feeling overwhelmed, introduce changes gradually, implementing two changes at a time over two months before adding more. This method can help reinforce positive habits and intentions for both you and your family.

Key Takeaways:

- ❖ The gut influences mood, immune function, and cognitive abilities, alongside digestion, acting like a second brain.

- ❖ Addressing gut health can positively impact behaviour and symptoms in autistic children by rewiring the brain through changing your child's environmental inputs and improving the metabolic health of their mitochondria.

- ❖ High sugar and ultra-high processed foods can disrupt the balance of gut bacteria, leading to inflammation and damage to the gut lining, contributing to Leaky Gut syndrome. Leaky Gut syndrome is very common for symptomatic autistic children.

- ❖ Gradually transitioning a child to a gluten-free and alpha/beta casein-free diet can help alleviate autism symptoms and improve gut health. But it requires patience and careful planning to ensure a smooth adjustment.

- ❖ Increasing dietary fibre and adding prebiotics and probiotics into your child's daily diet is crucial for maintaining gut health in autistic children.

- ❖ Maintaining a positive mindset throughout the process is essential.

Worksheet: Meal Ideas

1. What does your child usually eat?

2. How can we make some gluten-free alpha/beta casein-free substitutes for the meals your child is already eating?

3. Can you discreetly add more fibre or more plants to the meals your child is already eating?

4. Do you have an ethnic cuisine for your family?

5. Can you meal-prep any of these meals to make this more manageable for yourself?

6. When changing your child's meals, make a plan to change one meal at a time. Write your plan here. In a sustainable way, plan to change a second meal in 2-3 weeks time for your child, personalising this for how your child is finding these changes.

"It is too overwhelming to understand what the evolutionary mismatch we're in. People are suffering that don't need to be suffering, and if they understood that the modern world we're living in has taken us so off course with our health and we've got to start one by one, to figure out how to bring it back on course." – Dr Mindy Pelz

Chapter 4
Step 4: Take Down Toxins

In this chapter, we talk about the hidden chemicals in your home that can harm your child's health and brain development.

In today's world, we're surrounded by chemicals without even realising it. They've become part of our daily routines, like washing with soap, using sunblock, painting walls, cooking with non-stick pots, and using plastic lunch boxes.

These chemicals, even in small amounts, can interfere with your child's enzymes and hormone function, and create harmful molecules in their body called free radicals.[78] This will affect their metabolism and the health of their mitochondria.

What's more, when different low-dose chemicals from different sources mix in your child's body, they can react together in the body, causing different symptoms with the negative effects compounding over time. This is called bioaccumulation.[79]

All children have different potentials to detoxify their bodies. Autistic children can often have a lower potential to detoxify their bodies, so will have a higher dose of heavy metals found in their bodies. Hence a program to detoxify their bodies by supporting the four organs of detoxification[80] (gut, liver, kidneys, and skin) is essential to unlock your child's potential and will also improve their physical health.

Autism and Toxicity Evidence

There is a wealth of research which shows that children with autism spectrum disorder (ASD) typically have higher concentrations of heavy metals in their bodies compared to neurotypical children.

A systematic review (a research paper which evaluates the findings of lots of research papers) found that children with ASD had higher concentrations of cadmium, lead, arsenic, and mercury in their bodies compared to healthy control groups.[81] Another study reported higher concentrations of heavy metals in the baby teeth of children with autism compared to children without autism, suggesting that autistic children have been exposed to a higher amount of heavy metals while they are still in their mother's womb.

Every child will have a different ability to remove toxic heavy metals from their bodies. This explains why two children may have the exact same exposure to heavy metals, but one child will develop autism symptoms and the second child does not. However, it is clear that the higher the toxic load of heavy metals in a child's body, the greater impact on their physical health and brain health.

Heavy toxic metals in a person's body have not only been linked to autism symptoms developing, but also to other inflammatory health conditions developing, such as kidney failure, blood vessel damage, and different cancers.[82]

Are Low Levels Really That Bad?

You may be thinking, where are the laws and regulations to protect children and families from these heavy metals exposures?

Another sad realisation is that regulatory bodies in the UK and EU do look at the effect of these chemical compounds in our household and beauty products—but in isolation. So this means, perhaps the exposure of one chemical from a household product for a child may not necessarily be at a dangerous level, but children are being exposed to many different chemicals across their day/week from their environment. This is all getting absorbed in their body, and the bioaccumulation of different heavy metals in their bodies can react with each other to now cause dangerous neurological symptoms in your child.[83] Bioaccumulation refers to the gradual accumulation of substances, such as pollutants or toxins, in the tissues of humans building up over time.

Also, as these chemicals in our environment and homes is a relatively recent phenomenon in human history, the compounding effects in our human bodies is relatively unstudied.

What this means is that the heavy metal load in our bodies is increasing generationally. If a woman is pregnant with a baby girl, that baby's eggs for her entire life (the woman's future grandchildren) are already in that baby's tiny ovaries. So the things the woman eats and the toxins she is exposed to while pregnant will affect the quality of those eggs that are developing, and thus the physical health and brain health of her future grandchildren. This is why heavy metal toxicity's impact on people is getting worse with each generation.

Most scarily, a recent study in the journal Environment International found microplastics in developing foetuses while they are still in the womb.[84] This means toxins are accumulating in our children's bodies more with each generation, and goes to explain why neurological conditions like autism and its severity of symptoms are increasing with each generation.

Methylation

Exposure to toxic chemicals can disrupt the methylation cycle, which is vital for converting nutrients into energy and supporting various bodily functions. This cycle, often called the "B vitamins cycle," relies on B vitamins to enhance mood, energy, focus, detoxification, and immune response.[85] Research suggests a link between disrupted methylation and autism, with heavy metals and oxidative damage implicated in the condition.[86] Autistic children are likely to be undermethylated.[87] Minimising toxic exposure and detoxifying the body can help support a child's development and potential. I'll guide you through how to do this process step by step at home.

Your Child's Personal Hygiene and Beauty Products

Personal Care Products such as cosmetics, shampoos, sun lotion, nappy creams, nappy wipes, baby powder, children's toothpaste etc. are all modern inventions which children for millenia did not use. Often we think because we are washing off these chemicals from our bodies (e.g. shampoo) that they must be harmless. This isn't true. Our skin is a breathable organ, they push toxins out through sweat, but they also let toxins in.

These personal care products often contain chemicals, such as parabens and phthalates, which are known to disrupt hormones and affect brain development of children.[88] Phthalates exposure has been associated with learning and behavioural problems, including attention disorders, and can contribute to attention problems in children[89] such as in autism. Phthalates are known hormone disruptors, therefore will have an impact on the brain health of our children (and even their future fertility),[90] so exposure should be avoided in your home.[91]

Prevention is key; scan products using free apps like "Yuka"[92] or "Think Dirty"[93] to assess toxicity.

Replace harmful products with safer alternatives to detoxify and safeguard health. Paying attention to labels matters, as the products used affect not only immediate health but also of future generations.

I can definitely attest to the fact that now whenever I'm in a supermarket or drugstore, I have my apps out on my phone and I'm scanning any personal hygiene or beauty product before I take it home. Once you start scanning the products in your home, be prepared to feel horrified at what you have been putting on your child and on yourself.

Air

Some air fresheners release volatile organic compounds (VOCs) such as Formaldehyde or Benzene that can contribute to indoor air pollution, which can affect your child's lung health, and lead to poorer brain development.[94] Instead of using an air freshener, open your windows.

If you live in an area with high air pollution and are unable to move, filter the indoor air you breathe in by installing HEPA (high efficiency particulate arresting) filters in your bedrooms, living rooms, kitchen, and wherever else in your home that you and your children spend a lot of time in. Making this change in my family home has reduced everyone's hay fever symptoms too in the spring and summer time, and improved everyone's sleep quality.

If you have a wood-burning fireplace in your home, use an electric or gas fireplace instead, which will have fewer emissions. If you are unable to remove a wood-burning fireplace in your home, be sure that the circulation is very good, and that there are no leaks in the fireplace or flute.

Water

The World Health Organisation warns against any amount of lead in drinking water, while the UK set a limit of 10 ppb for tap water in 2013. A study by The Water Professor found 6.2% of UK samples exceeded this limit with 11.5% surpassing the EU's 5 ppb standard.[95] UK tap water also contains other harmful substances, like microplastics and trihalomethanes, linked to health issues like bladder cancer.[96]

Whole house carbon block filters ensure high-quality tap water, while products like the Water2 pod filter (backed by the University College London) filters out contaminants such as microplastics effectively.[97] I am not affiliated with this product but I can confirm our entire family is drinking more tap water since we've fitted our Water2 pod filter!

Black Mould

Sadly black mould is so common in homes in the UK.

The houses in this country are old, and are often poorly ventilated and insulated—prime conditions for black mould to grow fast. Exposure to black mould is dangerous for children and pregnant women due to the potential health effects of mycotoxins, cytokines, and volatile organic compounds (VOCs) produced by moulds.

Mycotoxins have been linked to a range of health problems, including causing inflammation in the brain and other parts of the body, which has been linked to a number of neurological disorders including autism.[98]

When I was pregnant with my son, like many people in the UK, I lived in a home full of black mould, so sadly I recognise that this exposure occurred for my son prenatally, and in his early years of life.

When I first learned about this, I cried blaming myself. But I am so grateful that there is a lot as parents that we can do now to detoxify and heal our children if this did happen to them. And showing yourself self-compassion for a situation you were in is so important to be able to move forward to helping yourself and your child.

To address the risk from black mould, check every area of your home for this, especially in kitchens and bathrooms, and fix any water leaks in your home. If your home does have a mould problem, a great solution, if you are able to do it, is to install a Positive Input Ventilation (PIV) unit in your home to blast clean air from the outside into your home and to insulate your homes carefully.

Some insulation, e.g. cavity wall insulation can be expensive to remove and can worsen household mould problems as they stop your home from "breathing," so they shouldn't be installed. Instead focus on double glazing windows and installing dehumidifiers and electric extractor fans where there are high humidity levels in certain rooms of your home, like bathrooms, kitchens, and basements.

Non-Stick Cookware and Food Packaging

The coating on non-stick pans can release perfluorinated chemicals when heated, which leaches into the food during the cooking process. A review of studies (a meta-analysis) by North Carolina State University concluded that these chemicals have been found widespread in human brains and that exposure during key development periods, such as during pregnancy and childhood, can negatively affect a child's behaviour and brain function long term.[99] Instead of using non-stick cookware, cook with stainless steel cookware, ceramic or glass cookware. Also, avoid purchasing food packaged in plastic or waxed liners. Throw out any plastic cooking utensils that you may have, and replace them with wooden utensils. Your food will also taste better with this change.

Plastic Food Containers

How many of us store our leftover foods in tubberware, have a plastic water bottle, and send our children to school with a plastic lunchbox? Many of these products contain known harmful chemicals such as bisphenol A (BPA) or phthalates, which over time can leach into food and drink. BPA can cause changes in a child's developing nervous system, leading to behavioural changes.[100] A safer alternative would be to store your leftover foods in glass containers, and to send your child to school with a steel lunchbox or an organic cotton insulated lunch box.

Cleaning Products

How many of us spray a product on our kitchen tables and worktops to make them shine after cleaning?

Many household cleaners in the UK contain chemicals like ammonia and bleach that can be harsh on our child's breathing systems when they breathe this in, and on their skin when they touch it. Swap out the cleaning products in your home using the recommendations in the Think Dirty app.A great product to swap with are Purdy & Figg cleaners; these products are non-toxic and readily available online.

Pesticides

Pesticides are often sprayed on our food before we eat it

during the farming phase. To decrease your pesticide exposure, purchase organic foods if possible or wash your fruit and vegetables with sodium bicarbonate before eating.

Additionally, we often all have sprays inside our homes to kill unwanted flies, mosquitoes, ants or other pests. These products all contain harmful chemicals such as: Organophosphates, Pyrethroids, Carbamates etc. These chemicals, called neurotoxins, are linked to problems in how children's brains develop. Exposure to them early in life can harm your child's nervous system and brain development.[101] Especially if that child is already epigenetically vulnerable to conditions such as autism. To reduce this risk, choose non-toxic brands such as "Ready Steady Defend Pesticide-Free Insect Killer Sprays."

Battery-Operated Toys and Plastic Toys with Electronic Features

Toys that require batteries often have electric circuit boards inside where lead solder may be used. If that toy becomes chipped or is frequently mouthed by the child, this can begin to leach lead inside the child's body. Even low levels of lead inside a child can cause typical autism symptoms, such as speech and language difficulties, increased aggression, hyperactivity, impulsivity, and concentration issues. Worryingly, The EU Toy Safety

Directive 2009 establishes maximum permissible limits for certain substances like lead in toys, instead of eliminating them entirely. This means that even with modern newly purchased toys, there is still a risk of lead leaching into a child's body. The risk is greater for older toys and toys purchased second-hand that may be in your home or your child's preschool.

To decrease this toxicity risk, declutter your home from any electric or battery-operated toys which may be chipped or which were purchased pre-2009. Choose wooden toys or natural cloth toys, which are made from brands known for producing non-toxic toys such as Hape or Uncle Goose.

Childrens' Clothes

Sadly in the UK, there are even toxic chemicals on our children's clothes!

Children's clothes are often dyed with colourants and sprayed with finishing agents to enhance its durability or wrinkle resistance. During the washing process, these chemicals can leach out of our washing machines and contaminate our water supply, and can irritate our children's skin.

To reduce this risk, purchase clothing without polybrominated diphenyl ethers (PBDEs). Choose clothes primarily made from natural fibres such as cotton, wool, hemp or silk, and wash all new clothing with a non-toxic laundry detergent before your child wears them for the first time to wash off these chemicals.

Furniture

Even the furniture in our homes are often sprayed with flame retardants, and can often contain a chemical called polybrominated diphenyl ethers (PBDEs). PBDEs are a class of chemicals that have been added to furniture foam, electronics, and other products to reduce their flammability. However, often when this furniture is exposed to heat, sunlight, or other factors, PBDEs can break down and be released into the air and dust. Inhalation or ingestion of these particles may lead to potential health risks in your child, including developmental and reproductive issues.

To prevent this, avoid spraying your furniture with "stain resistant" chemicals, which are toxic perfluorinated compounds. Instead, if furniture stains are a problem, buy non-fabric non-plastic furniture, e.g. leather or 100% organic cotton, linen blends, and wood. Or use covers which are easily washable.

House Paints

That fresh paint smell we love is caused by volatile organic compounds (VOCs), chemicals that evaporate at room temperature. Many companies now make low or no-VOC paints. The best option would be to use natural, earth-based paints and pigments if you find them and are willing to put up with a slightly less "polished" look.

Step-By-Step Detoxification of Your Child
Reading all of those chemicals can be quite a depressing read.

As we are so surrounded by these chemicals in our homes and our environments, it explains why autism spectrum disorder is a relatively modern epidemic, with rates of 2 children per 10,000 in the USA in the 1970s[102] to now be 1 in 36 children in 2023, according to the USA Centre of Disease Control.[103]

There are similar increasing rates in the UK too. This dramatic rate increase isn't just because there is more awareness of autism now. There have been widespread changes in our environment, which means autism is becoming more common. This heavy toxic load in our environment is a modern phenomenon, one that our human bodies were not evolved to deal with.

The first step to detoxify your child is to clean out your child's environment using the advice above. The next step would be to detoxify your child's body from any heavy metals that they have by supporting their four organs of detoxification.

These are the Gut, Liver, Kidney, and Skin. The way to detoxify your autistic child's body from heavy metals would be to follow these steps in order. If your child is very skinny, be careful before using this method.

You also might need to adjust each step to make the process slower, lasting more than two weeks, especially if your child isn't eating much. This helps prevent them from losing weight.

Again, ideally this change in diet should be performed under the supervision of a registered dietitian or paediatrician, but with NHS services being so overstretched, the wait could be very long before your child receives their first appointment!

Step 1: Supporting the Gut Function

Ideally, in the first two weeks, you should focus on helping your child eat a high-fibre, nil ultra-high processed food, and a nil pesticide diet.

In the past, humans ate between 100-150g fibre/day. Now it's typically 15g or less of fibre per day; only a tiny 4% of children in the UK are eating the recommended 25g of fibre a day.[104] This decrease in fibre consumption is similar for all children around the world as an ultra-high processed diet becomes more popular. This decrease in fibre consumption for a child will have an impact on their gut microbiome, and therefore impact their brain function because of the importance of the gut-brain bond. This pattern also helps explain why autism rates are increasing globally.

So the rules for these two weeks to support your child's gut function are:
- Aim for your child to eat a high-fibre diet (plant-based).
- Don't let your child eat: gluten, dairy, ultra-high processed foods, beef, chicken, farmed fish, non-organic (so non-pesticide laden) fruits and vegetables, artificial sweeteners, foods high in sugar and salt, and unfiltered water.
- For adults, alcohol and recreational drugs will also need to be avoided for this part of the detoxification process. In this book, I'm making the safe assumption that children will not have alcohol or recreational drugs as part of their diet.

What your child can eat:
- Fermented sourdough bread (as long as this has been fermented for at least 12 hours). I wanted to make it clear that none of the large supermarket chains in the UK who sell sourdough bread ferment their bread for at least

12 hours. So if you would like your child to eat sourdough bread as part of these two weeks or part of their regular diet, this would be something you will need to make fresh from home or purchase from a local baker.

- Free-range organic eggs can be eaten.
- Wild salmon or wild sardines are great fish sources. Tuna and swordfish are high in mercury so shouldn't be eaten. And factory farmed fish are high in chemicals such as PCBs and have a higher level of omega 6 which is very inflammatory. Hence should always be avoided.
- Cook only with Extra Virgin Olive Oil or Avocado oil or organic grass-fed ghee during these two weeks.
- Aim for your child to drink at least 1 litre of filtered water a day.
- Aim to have a source of fermented foods a day: kefir, kombucha, kimchi, sauerkraut or fermented vegetables. Even a teaspoon of this a day would be great for your child.
- Eat 100g of brassica foods a day. Brassicas are a class of cruciferous vegetables, such as turnips, broccoli, cabbage, kale and other bitter tasting vegetables. Aim to bake, braise or steam these foods. Avoid browning them as it can often mean generating more toxins from the frying pan during the cooking process.

- Use plenty of turmeric in your cooking, but avoid black pepper and cayenne pepper for these two weeks, which can increase gut permeability and slow down key liver detoxification enzymes respectively. Usually black pepper and cayenne pepper would be fine to include in your child's diet, but during these two weeks it should be avoided.

- Great fibre sources for your child are: flaxseed powder, pectin, alginate, nuts, seeds and fibre supplements, which are great at getting the recommended needed amount in children. For my recommendation on supplements see chapter 5. A high-fibre diet is really needed for this process, because as your child's body starts to dump all of those toxins from their body, their gut needs to have fibre in it to take these toxins out into their stools or they will simply get reabsorbed by their body system.

It is highly likely that your child will find this first week extremely difficult, as they withdraw from eating toxins that they are used to. In this time, their breath may smell, their energy may dip, and they may become crankier than normal. They may also experience a skin rash, headache, a runny or stuffy nose, and smellier stools or urine. These symptoms show that your child's body is releasing unwanted substances through every route possible.

But by the second week they should start to feel better and their autism symptoms will start to reduce. If the detox symptoms are increasing too much, then increase your child's intake of fibre through supplementation and berries, with a full glass of water three times a day to help absorb all of those toxins being dumped by their body. This way the toxins leave via the stools instead of through their body's other passages.

By understanding these symptoms, it should hopefully make the process less scary while it's happening. Additionally it will work to unlock your child's potential and help them reach their developmental milestones easier, so it will all be worth it.

Again, if you would prefer to slow down the rate of detoxification so that it happens over 4 weeks instead of 2 weeks, or with breaks in the stages, that is fine. This should be fine as long as your child is not eating any pesticide-heavy foods or ultra-high processed foods during their breaks, and as long as you have cleaned out their environment so that they aren't taking in as many chemicals from their environment anymore.

Example of meal and snack ideas which are autistic child-friendly for these two weeks are:

- Courgette omelettes or Courgette Gluten Free Pancakes
- Berry Almond Yogurt: Dairy-free coconut yoghurt with mixed berries and chopped almonds
- Baked Salmon Bites: Bite-sized wild-caught salmon with mild seasoning
- Kale Chips: homemade oven-baked kale chips
- Guacamole: homemade mashed avocado
- Garlic Broccoli with Lamb Chops: Lamb chops with lightly garlic-seasoned broccoli florets
- Brussels Sprouts Scramble: Scrambled eggs with chopped Brussels sprouts
- Strawberry Hemp Smoothie: Organic strawberry smoothie with hemp milk
- Chia Pudding: Chia seed pudding with berries
- Grilled Veggie "Rice": Grilled vegetables served with cauliflower "rice"
- Apple Almond Butter Snack: Sliced organic apple with almond butter
- Veggie Sticks with Hummus: Vegetable crudités with homemade hummus
- Lentil Patty: Lentil burger patty
- Sweet Potato Bites: Baked sweet potato wedges
- Steamed Broccoli Trees: Steamed broccoli florets

- Wild Salmon Fish Cakes: Mini wild salmon gluten-free fish cakes
- Fresh Fruit Medley: Assorted fresh fruit pieces
- Dairy-Free Milk: Almond or hemp or pea milk
- Gluten-Free Quinoa Pasta with Mini Grass-Fed Bison Meatballs
- French Toast: Sourdough French toast bites with mixed berries
- Sweet Potato Fries: Baked sweet potato fries
- Homemade gluten free chapatis with grass-fed ghee

Now for the serious question, how many of you were laughing at those meal suggestions?

To be honest, I get it.

My child didn't eat much of anything before when he was experiencing the worst of his autism symptoms. In these two weeks, just concentrate on getting as much of these food items in them as possible, even if just a few bites per meal, adding fibre supplements each day, and drinking plenty of filtered water in these two weeks. As long as you are avoiding harmful foods, drinking more water, and increasing your child's fibre intake, the detoxification process is taking place.

If your child's symptoms have already improved significantly after step 1, there is no need to proceed to step 2, 3 or 4.

Step 2: Supporting the Liver Function

Your child's liver eliminates many of the chemicals that modern life exposes us too. To support your child's liver function, for these two weeks, you should concentrate on increasing your child's nutrients and herbs to clean out their liver and improve the detoxification function of its enzymes.

This should be another 2-week process. In these two weeks, there is an emphasis on eating leafy green vegetables to get folic acid, and protein-rich and choline-rich foods such as eggs. Foods rich in B vitamins (wholegrains) and vitamin C (peppers, cabbage, citrus foods) are also important in these two weeks, as well as eating a daily high multivitamin supplement and fish oil supplement (see recommendations for this in chapter 6).

Foods to eat during these two weeks to support the Liver Function are:
- Eggs, especially the yolk part which is high in choline, 5x a week if possible
- Cooked beans or lentils (high in fibre and in sulphur supporting liver function) 4x a week

- Wild sardines, anchovies or small mackerel 4x a week
- Sunflower seeds and sesame seeds
- Cooked broccoli, cabbage, brussel sprouts, asparagus or other green leafy vegetables
- Artichokes eaten every other day with lemon juice and organic extra virgin olive oil
- Avocado or walnuts every other day
- Whole grain steel-cut oats (high in fibre, trace minerals and B vitamins)
- Two oranges, lemons or limes a week
- Dandelion dried roots supplement or fresh steamed dandelions from pesticide-free lawns
- Turmeric
- Fish Oil and Multivitamin supplements everyday (see chapter 6 for recommended brands)

Example of meal and snack ideas which are autistic child-friendly for these two weeks are:
- Scrambled eggs with refried beans
- Sliced oranges
- Sourdough toast
- Sliced apples
- Homemade porridge with gluten-free, steel-cut oats with cinnamon apples, chopped walnuts, and sunflower seeds

- Turkey chilli with millet (gluten-free grain) and steamed kale
- Apple-cabbage salad
- Steamed artichokes
- Hummus with sliced peppers
- Garlic-sesame broccoli with walnut sauce
- Quinoa porridge with diced apples, chopped walnuts, and a touch of cinnamon
- Sardines with lemon
- Dilled cauliflower
- Broccoli and Brussels sprouts stir-fry with sesame sauce
- Steamed artichoke with lemon hummus dip
- Black bean and red quinoa soup
- Steamed greens with orange butter
- Avocado salad

Again, if you are laughing at the above menu, then feel free to modify it, as long as it remains dairy-free, gluten-free, high in eggs, high in artichokes, high in vitamin C, and contains some of the foods from the "Foods to eat during these two weeks" section for the Liver above.

As above, if toxins are being released too quickly by your child's body, they will feel sicker and their energy will be lower. So you can slow down this stage as well for your child. And remember, if your child's symptoms have already improved significantly after steps 1 and 2, then there is no need to proceed to steps 3 or 4.

Step 3: Supporting the Kidney Function

The main function of your child's kidneys is to filter toxins from their blood. To do that job properly, it requires that adequate blood flow is passing through the kidneys everyday. To ensure this, during these two weeks, your child should eat a diet high in filtered water, avoiding excessive protein, and avoiding excessive phosphates in their diet.

Kidneys are very vulnerable to long term damage from toxin exposure. Improving their function is critical for toxin elimination and for reducing your child's autism symptoms. During these two weeks, the process will focus on improving the blood supply to the kidneys to promote their function. To do this, include as much of the following in your child's daily diet:

- 1 litre of filtered water a day
- Homemade fresh Beetroot juice
- Blueberries
- Dark chocolate (70% or greater, low in refined sugar and without heavy metals in it)
- Turmeric
- Gingko Biloba
- Ginger
- Gotu Kola herbs

- Daily multivitamin

Remember if toxins are being released too quickly by your child's body, they will feel sicker and their energy will be lower so you can slow down this stage as well for your child. Also, if your child's symptoms have already improved significantly after steps 1, 2 and 3, then there is no need to proceed to step 4.

Step 4: Supporting the Skin Function

This is another two-week stage. To help your child's skin to sweat out toxins, concentrate on having your child perform high-intensity exercise outdoors everyday where they are sweating for at least one hour. In these two weeks, your child can also have infrared saunas for 30 minutes a day to support their skin's detoxification function.

The Detoxification Stages

Many clients have found relief from autism symptoms through these detox steps. As a parent who has followed them, I understand the challenges but can confirm their effectiveness. Witnessing your child's transformation is incredibly rewarding and is so much better than watching your child struggle indefinitely.

As a parent doing these steps myself, I can definitely confirm they are tough. But with persistence, filtered water, and lots of fibre, this all does work to detoxify your child. Experiencing the transformation firsthand, seeing your child for the first time who is now relaxed, giving eye contact, and can speak, there is nothing like it as a parent. You definitely do not take it for granted.

You don't need to complete all four stages at once; many see significant improvements with just the first step for their child. In today's toxin-filled world, minimising exposure and detoxifying benefits everyone's health. For many of my clients who complete these steps with their child, they have said that it has helped with their symptoms from a wide range of conditions, e.g. for rheumatoid arthritis, rosacea, kidney dysfunction, migraines, and other symptoms, while boosting their energy levels. So it may be worth you joining your child with these detoxification steps while your child does this.

Key Takeaways:

❖ The modern world is filled with chemicals that permeate our daily lives, from cleaning products to personal care items, furniture, and even children's toys. These chemicals, though often unseen, can have profound effects on our children's health and development.

❖ Even low doses of modern chemicals can disrupt enzyme function, hormone levels, and create harmful molecules in the body, impacting metabolic health. Children on the autism spectrum may have a reduced ability to detoxify their bodies, leading to higher levels of heavy metals in their bodies and exacerbating their symptoms.

❖ Toxic chemicals can bioaccumulate in the body. This can disrupt the methylation cycle, affecting energy production, mood, and immune function. Poor methylation, coupled with compromised gut health, can lead to various health symptoms including autism. Supporting the body's detoxification process—focusing, in order, on the gut, liver, kidneys and skin—is crucial for reducing heavy metal toxicity and unlocking your child's potential.

❖ It's important to pay attention to how your child's body responds to the detoxification process. If they start feeling sicker or have lower energy levels, you can slow down the detoxification stages. Or if your child's autism symptoms have already improved significantly after completing certain steps, there may be no need to proceed to the next stage. Remember, every child is different, and it's essential to tailor the detoxification process to suit their individual needs and responses.

"You are not what you eat, you are what you absorb, digest and excrete."

–Shim Ravalia

Part 3:
Cognition and
Connection

Chapter 5
Step 5: Solve With Supplements

It is very important that these steps are completed in order before starting any supplementation. If your child's body is still high in toxins or they still have a leaky gut, then this can interfere with their methylation process. This means that any supplements they start taking will not be absorbed properly, and will therefore be ineffective, and the child will be making very expensive urine.

Value of Supplementation
First of all, if a child has a perfectly healthy organic balanced healthy diet, great sleep, plenty of outdoor exercise every single day, then they may not need to take any supplements.

However, there are very few people in this country who do live and eat like that, although that is something we should all be aiming for. In the UK, most children are generally low on Omega 3, Fibre and Vitamin D3 etc., and so would benefit from taking a daily supplement.

The best way to think of supplements would be as an insurance policy. So just in case your child is not eating everything that they need to optimise their physical growth and brain function, supplementation can be effective and will usually have very few side effects, if any.

The supplements that I think all autistic children (and most likely their parents!) would benefit from taking everyday are:

- A quality multivitamin liquid supplement
- An Omega 3/Fish oil supplement
- A fibre supplement everyday

After a child starts taking a good quality multivitamin and omega-3/fish oil every day, it usually takes about six months of starting this for their body to reach their optimal levels of its needed nutrients.

Overall the choice of supplements should definitely be guided from the results of your child's blood test, taken as part of step 2 of the 7-Step Autism Action Plan. In all my years working with clients, I have not seen the blood test result of a single autistic child which shows they are not deficient in anything. So there will definitely be benefits from supplementation.

I really would like to stress that parents should not skip to this section of the book as a shortcut or as an easy answer to eliminate their child's autism symptoms. There is an order to this process, and if your child is not methylating properly because their gut lining is damaged due to inflammation, or because of an increase in heavy metals inside their bodies, then no supplement will help them. It'll be passed right through your child and it won't be absorbed. Your child's body's ability to absorb is a lot less when their gut is inflamed inside or compromised. Hence do not skip steps 1-4 of the 7-Step Autism Action Plan!

Daily Supplements Recommended for All Autistic Children

A high-quality liquid multivitamin provides essential vitamins and minerals crucial for your child's immune system and growth. Taking this everyday ensures your child will be receiving all of the necessary nutrients vital for optimal brain development. It is well known that vitamin deficiencies can lead to illness, making a daily multivitamin a valuable tool in preventing immune-related issues. This is particularly important if your child is a fussy eater. As a general rule of thumb, liquid forms of supplements are absorbed better by the body than gummy forms, especially by people with poorer gut health. Hence if you are able to encourage your child to take a liquid multivitamin instead of a gummy multivitamin, this may be more effective.

Omega 3 Supplements or a Fish Oil supplement is so important to help a child's speech develop, reduce their hyperactivity,[106] decrease inflammation in the brain, improve sleep, mood, and attention, and reduce aggression.[107] Autistic children can generally have an Omega 3 index less than 1%, whereas children with ADD/ADHD can have an Omega index of less than 3%. An optimal Omega 3 index is between 8-12%.

After your child starts taking a daily supplement, depending on your child's original omega 3 index level, it can take up to 6 months for this to build up in your child to a baseline level where their potential will be unlocked dramatically. If your child is vegetarian/vegan, then you can look for an algae-based omega 3 supplement for your child to take. A good omega 3 supplement is one which contains a high dose of EPA and DHA within it.

The majority of people in the UK are low in fibre and have a daily fibre intake of 18g. A child's fibre intake should be 25g per day.[108] The value of taking a supplement high in fibre is that it really improves a person's gut health, moves toxins out of their body, and can help ease constipation, which is a very common symptom for autistic children. Within the market there are many vegan, tasteless, odourless, and suitable-for-children fibre supplements, which are safe for everyday use. So find one that works for your family.

Alongside my son, I make sure that I take a multivitamin, an Omega 3 supplement, and a fibre supplement everyday. For years I just purchased this for my children, because as a parent they were my priority. However when my daughter was 9 months old, I was admitted into hospital with kidney stones and needed an operation to remove them. The time away from both my children did not help their wellbeing or consistency, and from then on I decided that part of making my children's health a priority, means I needed to make my own health a priority too.

So I started adding to my daily routine to give myself my supplements whenever I give my children theirs in the morning. I have noticed a boost in my immunity and alleviation of my previous brain fog and fatigue since I started this new routine. For my children, since taking these daily supplements, their sick days at nursery have at least halved, which makes for a very happy parent!

To find specific product recommendations for these supplement types for children, please scan the QR code below. This will take you to a downloadable table recommending specific products for yourself and for your child.

It's worth noting that for many families, daily supplements like a liquid multivitamin, omega-3, and fibre are sufficient to significantly improve their child's autism symptoms. These, combined with the diet and lifestyle changes described in steps 1-4, often bring about positive results for families without needing additional supplements.

However I have listed the names of some other supplements which can help with specific autistic challenges. Please keep in mind that these specific supplements are not a quick fix – the key to unlock your autistic child's potential is in the whole 7-Step Autism Action Plan.

But if after six months of making these diet and lifestyle changes consistently for your child, if your child still faces challenges with their autism symptoms, you might consider the supplements mentioned below.

Specific supplements which can help with speech and language difficulties include: Cod Liver Oil, Vitamin B12, Thiamin, Leucovorin, 5-MTHF, Acetyl L Carnitine, Dimethylglycine, Carnosine, Namenda, Galantamine, Magnesium bath flakes, Theanine, Phosphatidylcholine and Phosphatidylserine.

Specific supplements which can help your child get out of consistent Fight-Flight-Freeze modes are: Valerian root, Ashwagandha, Rhodiola Ginseng, Green Tea Extract, Ginseng and GABA calming.

Supplements which can help a child with their anxiety include: Vitamin D3, Valerian Root Extract, Magnesium bath flakes, GABA Calming and Theanine.

Supplements which can help your child fall asleep and stay asleep include bathing with Magnesium Flakes, 5-HTP, Benadryl, GABA Calming and Theanine.

If your child wakes up very angry, they may have low blood sugar. Often giving a glass of apple juice in the morning straight away can correct this for them, or giving them an early protein-heavy breakfast, perhaps even last night's dinner for breakfast (brinner!). Otherwise supplements which can help to raise your child's blood sugar if they are a particularly hangry child are: chromium, berberine, cinnamon, and nutmeg.

Specific supplements to raise your child's serotonin if they are depressed or low include taking Saffron, Vitamin B6 or 5-HTP.

For a child who is always worried, rigid, inflexible, argumentative, and oppositional, then giving 5-HTP to build serotonin in them can calm down the hyper frontal part of their brain. Then after the 5-HTP, Vitamin B6 and saffron supplements can be given to the child. Saffron is the happy herb and it improves memory and depression symptoms. In fact there are over 20 randomised controlled studies which show that saffron is equally effective to Prozac and Zoloft in treating depression.[109] Supplements to increase your child's focus include Cod Liver Oil, Rhodiola, Ashwagandha, Ginseng, Green tea extract, L Tyrosine, L Theanine, Taurine, Omega 3, Cinnamon and Nutmeg.

It is important to realise that not all supplement companies are made equal to each other. Therefore you must look at their formulations to check if they are toxin-free. You can do this by scanning the barcode of these products with the Yuka app, which works for food sources too.

Supplements definitely do not cure autism. What they can do is help support the mechanism that as a parent you are trying to target, like sleep or focus.

If you are trying these extra supplements for your child (after already completing steps 1-4 of the 7-Step Autism Action Plan), then it's important to have a curious scientific mindset. You have to ask yourself, is this supplement working? If not, then stop it and don't stack supplements on top of eachother. Continue to journal daily with what you've done and record how your child's behaviour is that day. This will help you determine if your child exhibits any behaviour or symptom changes—or not—since starting this supplement.

Sleep

Many autistic children do have a problem with sleep. This has become an increasing modern problem, as we are surrounded by more blue light, gadgets, and dopamine-addicting distractions than ever before.

Before trying the specific sleep supplements mentioned above, make sure your child's sleep hygiene is good. Try to turn off their gadgets at least two to four hours before they sleep, and add blue light blockers on the gadgets that they are using throughout the day. Blue light blocks melatonin production in their body, so will make it harder for your child to go to sleep. Ensure that their bedroom has blackout blinds across all their windows.

Using a red light watt bulb in their room before they go to bed is a great idea because red light stimulates the secretion of melatonin, and can help make the child sleepy. Red light also improves muscle gain and sleep quality.

Another great tip is to make sure your child is out in the morning light as soon as they wake up (even if it's cold outside!). There is something special about the first light of the morning to reset your child's body clock to help them fall asleep at night and stay alert during the day.

For autistic children who go to sleep on time but wake up at midnight or odd hours in the morning, look at their sleep hygiene. Ensure that they are not having sugar before bedtime and that they are well fed three hours before bedtime.

Also, if you have a child who consistently wakes up at 2:00 a.m, then ask yourself how are you putting the child asleep? Are you rocking them asleep? Every child has three to four sleep cycles at night, if the only way to initiate sleep for them is to be rocked or watching TV before bed, then that is what the child is going to want and need to put themselves to sleep again in the middle of the night too.

If this sounds like your child, then your child does not have a melatonin problem—they have a sleep hygiene problem. Additionally, you should not nurse a child to sleep, or rock them to sleep or give them a bottle to sleep. Otherwise they will need this every three to four hours like clockwork through their sleep cycles. Learning how to fall asleep independently each night is a skill that children need to learn by themselves.

Potty Training

Autistic children can often struggle with bowel control. If the child is older than 4 years old but is still using nappies during the day or night, or unable to use the toilet for poo, then we would usually say that the child is developmentally delayed for this skill.

There can be three key reasons why your child may be struggling with potty training:

1. It could be that the child's gut and brain are not communicating properly, so the child does not realise that they have a full bladder or bowel. This would also apply if a child is older than 4 years old but they are still wet every night.
2. The child has a lot of constipation so they can not relieve themselves.
3. Or it could be linked to anxiety, so that when the child is feeling anxious (even in unprovoked situations), they are having an accident.

For the child who is still wet at night or having a lot of poo/pee accidents, this means their gut and brain are not talking to each other properly. To resolve this, usually cleaning the child's diet as shown in step 3 and detoxifying their environment as seen in step 4 will help. If this hasn't helped the child and the child is having a lot of accidents, or is still not dry overnight, this could indicate a yeast infection. In these cases, it would be best to get their gut tested by a specialist, like The Gut Intuition company in London.

For the child who is unable to poop in the toilet because they have a lot of constipation, a high-fibre diet and soluble-fibre supplements which are part of step 3 and step 4 of the program should help resolve this. But if your child still avoids going to the bathroom even after doing the first 4 steps of this program, it might be because they're afraid it will hurt.

In this case, talking to your child's GP about using an enema or a stool softener could be helpful. These can make it more comfortable for your child to go to the bathroom and teach them that it's okay and comfortable to relieve themselves like this.

Lastly, if your child is in the third case where they are having accidents when they are in a stressful or anxious situation, then the next steps of cerebellum stimulation and emotional literacy as part of this book will benefit these children.

Key Takeaways:

❖ It's crucial to prioritise detoxification steps before considering supplementation for your child. High toxin levels can interfere with the body's ability to absorb supplements, rendering them ineffective and costly.

❖ While a perfectly balanced diet and lifestyle are ideal, most children, including autistic ones, may benefit from supplements due to dietary deficiencies. Supplements should be viewed as an insurance policy to ensure optimal growth and brain function.

❖ A quality multivitamin liquid, Omega 3/Fish oil, and a fibre supplement are recommended for all autistic children to support the immune system, growth, brain function, and gut health.

❖ Supplements do not cure autism but can support specific mechanisms targeted for improvement, such as sleep, focus, and mood. It's essential to adopt a curious scientific mindset, journal daily observations, and not stack supplements without monitoring their effectiveness.

Chapter 6
Step 6: Charge the Cerebellum

"When your brain works right, you work right."
- Dr. Daniel Amen

For autistic individuals, the cerebellum (an area at the lower back part of the brain) is commonly smaller in size and is underdeveloped compared to neurotypical children. The cerebellum is commonly known as "the brain's brain." Although it makes up only 10% of the overall size of the brain, it has 80% of the brain's connections within it.[110] The cerebellum "learns"—by creating the automatic skills and processes that happen without us having to consciously think about them.

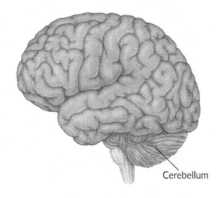

Cerebellum

The cerebellum is the part of the brain that helps with movements and thinking, so having a smaller cerebellum will cause problems with moving, balance and thinking skills.

It can also affect how well autistic individuals will pay attention, use language, or handle their emotions. These are all skills that autistic individuals will typically struggle with. As the cerebellum is smaller in autistic individuals, there is an unproven theory that this is one of the reasons why autistic individuals stim, to try and activate this area of their brain.

Fortunately, like every area of the brain, using neuroplasticity, a person's cerebellum can be grown, moulded, and rewired with intentional practice. A program which aims to unlock the potential within your autistic child must include a focus on growing their cerebellum in size. This can be done in a variety of ways, and the best ways would include all of the following.

Equine/Horse Therapy

It is well known that working with horses and horse riding can have therapeutic benefits for autistic children.

First of all the relationship between a rider and a horse is one full of bonding and trust, so it boosts the love hormone oxytocin, which is an essential hormone to help learn new skills faster.

Second of all, and most relevant to this section of the book, the level of coordination required to sit on a horse is different from almost everything else a person does. Equine therapy would stimulate and grow a child's cerebellum, which will improve their learning capabilities and unlock their potential.

Equine therapy has been proven to offer clinically significant reductions in disability in the areas of communication, perception, attention, and emotion regulation for people with autism. It has also been reported to improve sensory integration, reduce hyperactivity, and decrease impulsivity in individuals with autism.[111]

Follow-up studies on the effects of horse therapy found significant long-term benefits for autistic children, including sustained improvements in social communication and word fluency. Equine therapy can also help children with autism by reducing symptoms of irritability and hyperactivity, as well as improving communication and building emotional bonds. It does all of this through growing the size of the cerebellum.

For my son, I aimed to take him on a pony-riding lesson once every month. This was often enough for him to expect it and not forget that he had previously been, but not so often enough that it became a pricey burden! Being around the ponies definitely had a calming effect on him, and there really is a special bond of trust between a horse and their rider.

Barefoot Walking

For millennia, humans did not wear shoes and were always barefoot. It may be surprising to learn that there are a similar number of muscles in our hands and in our feet,[112] but the level of dexterity and strength in our hands for most people is so much greater than for their feet. These muscles in a person's feet can be trained and grown through barefoot walking, and this would also stimulate and grow their cerebellum too.

A person's feet can take in a wide variety of sensory information, which can benefit their nervous system functioning and grow a person's cerebellum. In addition, barefoot walking has another benefit of grounding/earthing. All humans naturally build up a charge inside our bodies, which can be discharged naturally through bare-feet walking on sand, grass, or soil.[113] This process, called grounding/earthing, can help reset a child's nervous system and stress responses, and bring about a calming effect for an individual. The benefits of daily grounding/earthing for autistic individuals is well known in scientific literature, and I always ask my clients to commit to at least 5 to 30 minutes a day of this completely free treatment.[114] My clients will often report their child will appear calmer and sleep better on the days that they have done grounding or earthing that day. The time in nature is also very beneficial in relaxing the child's nervous system from the fight/flight/freeze system.

Avoid Noise-Cancelling Headphones

It is very common to see autistic individuals walk around with noise-cancelling headphones. For my child, I was advised to purchase this for him as he had sensory overwhelm to sound. This never sat right to me, as my son also had poor balance, lacked social skills, and he was non-verbal. It seemed to me that giving my son noise-cancelling headphones would be treating a symptom of autism (sensory overwhelm from sound) but would not address the cause of autism, which is partly from having a smaller cerebellum size. Additionally, I thought it would make his social skills, speech, and balance worse (as a person's balance system is inside their ears). Thankfully I didn't purchase noise-cancelling headphones, but instead drew my attention to creating a lifestyle program for my child, which would grow his cerebellum.

Martial Arts, Tennis and Dancing

These are great coordination sports for people to engage in to grow a person's cerebellum. As long as there is no risk of head injuries occurring, so make sure to double check the philosophy of the karate course before enrolling your child. Martial arts, tennis, and dancing all involve coordination of both sides of the body, increases a person's muscle tone, strength and mindfulness and activates their cerebellum helping it to grow in size. There have been many randomised control trials which show how beneficial martial arts, tennis and dancing is for autistic people.[115] Some of these benefits include: improved mental awareness and calmness, increased mental awareness, fostering calmness and enhancing cognitive function.

Neurofeedback

This is a potentially game-changing treatment for children with autism. How it works is that a practitioner will put sensors on a child's head and measure their brain wave activity. It will then provide feedback to the child's brain in a non-invasive way, through an activity like watching a movie, and change the inputs the child is receiving by changing the volume and picture size of the movie. Another activity sample is through touch, like when a child is holding a vibrating teddy. It is based on the premise that the brain will try to make sense of the information it is receiving, similar to how a person can still understand and read sentences where all the vowels are removed.

So from these specific sound, sight, and touch inputs, the brain will change and rewire to make sense of the information it receives from the movie. The practitioner will devise a program to strengthen different areas of the brain associated with the symptoms that you would like to work on, like speech or sleep or potty training through growing the different areas of the brain, including the cerebellum.[116] After twenty sessions of neurofeedback, the effects are usually permanent, and reduce the autism symptoms that you would like the child not to have, helping to unlock their potential.[117]

Cereskills

This is a UK-based company that provides an assessment for a child to see which areas of the brain needs growth. It is aimed for children aged 7+. Cereskills (formerly known as Zing Performance) will then provide a framework of personalised coordination exercises for the child to do everyday for 20 minutes, which will activate and grow their cerebellum.

Usually children will finish their program within 6-9 months, and parents report having a calmer child, a child with better emotional control, memory and coordination, and even reading skills. Central to reading is having strong eye tracking muscles to be able to read sentences and paragraphs.

Therefore strengthening the cerebellum through a Cereskills program will improve lots of different areas of development for children.

There is so much we can do as parents to help unlock our child's potential. As part of doing this, it must include a program to grow their cerebellum, and the effects of doing this will be far reaching.

Key Takeaways:

❖ The cerebellum, located at the back of the brain, plays a crucial role in coordinating movements and cognitive processes. Despite comprising only 10% of the brain's size, it houses 80% of the brain's connections, earning it the nickname "the brain's brain."

❖ Autistic individuals typically have a smaller cerebellum compared to neurotypical individuals. This smaller size contributes to challenges in movement, balance, attention, language usage, and emotional regulation— common difficulties faced by autistic individuals.

❖ Intentional practices can aid in growing and rewiring the cerebellum. Activities such as equine therapy, barefoot walking, martial arts, tennis, dancing, and neurofeedback can stimulate the cerebellum, improving coordination, sensory integration, and emotional regulation.

❖ Structured programs like martial Arts, dance, horse therapy, or Cereskills offer personalised coordination exercises aimed at growing the cerebellum. These programs have shown promising results in enhancing various areas of development, including speech, emotional control, memory, coordination, and reading skills, ultimately helping your child reach their developmental milestones and unlock their potential.

❖ By focusing on growing the cerebellum, parents can play a proactive role in supporting their children with autism, leading to far-reaching improvements in their overall well-being and development.

Chapter 7
Step 7: Empower Emotions

"Emotional intelligence is a key factor in our success, relationships, and overall happiness. It is the ability to understand and manage our own emotions and to recognise and influence the emotions of others."
- Daniel Goleman

In this chapter, I'm going to talk about how to implement the last step in the 7-Step Autism Action Plan, which is Emotional Empowerment. This aims to help parents teach the skill of emotional literacy to their autistic child. A growth mindset means that a person's skill levels are not fixed, but all skills can be learned and developed through practice and intentional teaching.

Sadly in this world, when someone thinks of an "autistic adult" or "autistic child," they think of someone who struggles with communication skills and with relationships. Like many other millions of people in this world, I watched Robert Waldinger's Ted Talk "What Makes a Good Life? Lessons from the Longest Study On Happiness" years ago, well before I became a Mum. What I learned was that the healthiest person, physically and emotionally, is the one who has the most social connections, informally and formally, and that these relationships are protective for a person's physical health and brain health.

Watching that Ted Talk at a young age made me realise a new dream for myself and my children, one rich in social connection. Knowing that autistic individuals struggle with recognising their own emotions and of other people made me create a program of emotional literacy for my child. Once my child and my clients' children begin to have words, we begin a program of building up their emotional vocabulary.

I have had an emotionally tumultuous life and I first had clinical depression when I was in my early twenties. I had all of the horrible symptoms, and I did the things that we are advised to do by our GPs: I started taking antidepressants and began counselling (no one asked me about my gut health, told me about saffron or tested my vitamin D levels!). I completed months of counselling and I only began to turn a corner when I learned the name of the feeling that was ruminating inside of me, which was "rejection."

Once I was able to recognise and name that feeling, I began to process it and make strides.

That experience was transformative for me, so when I designed a curriculum for my son to develop his emotional literacy, I created flash cards and books which would label feelings and give him that vocabulary (and of course I made sure the word rejection was on one of the flash cards!).

As part of my program to develop my clients' children's emotional skills, I ask the parent to practise the following with their child:

Play a game of naming emotions from flash cards, and for the child to guess the name of the emotion that face is showing
I believe giving small children this vocabulary is a gift to them for the rest of their lives, for the relationship they have with themselves and the relationship they have with others.

Read plenty of books which teach emotional literacy and relationship skills

Some of my favourites to recommend are the Mini Monsters series: "Can I Be The Best?" And "Can I Play?" These definitely depict real life experiences that children will have on the playground, and are so great at naming those emotions. Other recommendations are, "Let's Talk About Body Boundaries, Consent and Respect" by Jayneen Sanders and "Hey Little Ant" by Philip Moose. Fortunately there are a lot more choices with books around this subject than there were when I was growing up.

Encourage your child to say "I feel... when... because..." statements

For example, "*I feel* sad *when* Daddy goes to work *because* I miss him" or "*I feel* scared *when* the lights are turned off *because* I think there is a monster in the room." Encouraging an expression of this emotion gets it out of a child's nervous system and helps to improve their communication skills, which will help improve all of their relationship-building skills as a child and as an adult. Who else has heard this a million times: "Communication is the key to every good relationship."

Role play is incredibly useful

Whenever a difficult situation occurs for your child in real life which they are having trouble with, use dolls to role play that situation at home, explaining all the feelings that each doll is having in the situation. Then give your child the dolls to role-play that situation themselves as many times as they want to over the next few weeks. Feel free to let them release any cathartic emotions they are having with their dolls at that time too. This was some game-changing advice that I received for my own son and that I teach to my clients. One of my clients lives separately from her ex-husband, and her ex-husband will drop in to see his 4-year old and 3-year old daughters every few months or so. This really confuses the youngest child in particular, and her behaviour will usually go really bad, with lots of tantrums for the next week or so after a visit from her dad. Since the mother implemented this technique after her ex-husband visits, her daughter has become calmer, understands the situation more, and is able to express her emotions through this role-playing game with the dolls. It has been a game changer!

Teach your child self-regulation exercises, like deep breathing when feeling strong emotions

When teaching your child deep breathing, make sure to teach the child to take a longer exhale out of the mouth, and a shorter inhale through the nose (4 seconds in, 8 seconds out). This breathing technique will activate a child's parasympathetic system, so will help them get out of the fight/flight/freeze modes of the sympathetic nervous system.

Teach your child mindfulness

This can be done in a variety of ways, including mindfulness listening when outdoors or mindful eating. But one of my favourite effective ways include teaching your child how to do a "body scan." You can do this by having your child lie down comfortably and focus on the different parts of their body, starting from their toes and moving up to their head. Encourage them to notice any sensations, tension, or relaxation in each body part, to be aware of this and to give them this vocabulary. To change anything, self-awareness has to be the first step.

Another self-regulation exercise to teach your child is the 54321 grounding exercise

This is great to practise when your child is feeling anxious or stressed. The 5-4-3-2-1 exercise involves using their senses to bring your child's focus back to the present moment to ground themselves. Guide your child throughout by counting down from 5 to 1, prompting them to engage each sense along the way. For example:

    a. "Let's start by looking around and finding 5 things you can see. Take your time to notice each thing and describe it to me."

b. "Now, listen carefully and name 4 things you can hear. It could be the sound of birds chirping, cars passing by, or even your own breathing."

c. "Next, touch 3 things around you. Pay attention to how they feel. Are they rough, smooth, warm, or cold?"

d. "Take a deep breath and notice 2 things you can smell. It could be the scent of flowers, food cooking, or even the fresh air."

e. "Finally, notice 1 thing you can taste. It could be the taste of toothpaste from brushing your teeth or a lingering flavour from a recent meal."

After this exercise you will notice your child should feel calmer.

Modelling

As with teaching your child any new behaviour, you must model the above techniques when you feel yourself getting dysregulated too as a parent. Don't be surprised if your child reminds you to take deep breaths or to do the 5-4-3-2-1 grounding technique if they see you becoming dysregulated. If your child is reminding you to do this behaviour, this should be considered as a success in my eyes.

Make sure you are practising self-love and self-care behaviours too as caring for children, let alone an autistic child/children is demanding

Parental stress is contagious to their children and to other people around them. So as well as encouraging emotional literacy and self-regulation skills in your child, include them in your daily routine too. My favourite way to practise self-love and self-care is to have a habit of journaling every night. This is where I just write down all my own feelings (positive, neutral, and negative) and how I feel my day went everyday. Through this practice, I am releasing these emotions from my nervous system. Walking in nature and practising mindfulness is another great practice to include in your daily/weekly routine too.

Another fabulous way to develop your child emotionally, which isn't easily available to everyone, hence I have included it at the end, is to expand your family with a pet dog or a pet cat

As I explained in an earlier chapter, autistic children can often have a special bond with animals. They help the child release oxytocin, the love hormone which helps speed up their learning, and helps them if they are feeling dysregulated. Caring for a pet dog can help children develop empathy, as they learn to consider the needs of their pet and recognise non-verbal cues, which can also be applied to understanding human emotions.

They can also reduce a child's stress levels, and caring for pets can give children a sense of purpose and boost their self-esteem. If you are able to expand your family with a well-trained pet dog or pet cat, you should definitely consider it, as they would give more back to your family than they take.

Another interesting insight is that self-love, self-confidence, self-worth, and gut health are all connected. The more self-care practices you put in place for yourself and for your child, the more positive impact it will have on your gut health and your child's gut health, and both of your overall well-being.

There is growing evidence that the more you practise self-love, the less stress and tension you will experience, which takes the pressure off of your gut, nervous system, and overall, your entire body.

Key Takeaways:

- ❖ Having strong relationships and social connections is the most important factor to predicting a person's long term physical and mental health. Teaching children emotional vocabulary and literacy is essential to help them develop the skills needed to form healthy social connections when they are adults. Naming and recognising emotions helps children understand and manage their feelings better.

- ❖ Engage children in activities, such as naming emotions from flashcards, reading books on emotional literacy, and role-playing difficult situations with dolls to enhance their emotional intelligence.

- ❖ Teach children self-regulation techniques, like deep breathing and mindfulness, to help them manage strong emotions and reduce stress. The 5-4-3-2-1 grounding exercise is particularly effective for calming anxiety and bringing focus back to the present moment.

- ❖ Parents should model these techniques themselves to reinforce their importance and effectiveness. Practising self-love and self-care is crucial for both parents and children to reduce stress levels and promote overall well-being and gut health.

❖ Consider expanding your family with a pet, as they can provide emotional support and teach empathy.

"You are always one decision away from a totally different life." - Eddie Pinero

Conclusion

The 7-Step Autism Action Plan puts the control and power back into your hands as a parent, and gives you the power to help your autistic child unlock their potential, and start reaching their developmental milestones sooner.

Step 1: Optimise Oxytocin helps build the parent-child bond and increases your child's oxytocin levels to provide the right environment for them to learn new skills faster.

Step 2: Break Down Blood helps you to exclude any other possible medical reason to explain their current symptoms and discover any nutritional deficiencies your child may have.

Step 3: Grasp the Gut-Brain Bond explores the typical gut microbiome seen in autism, its influence on brain health and behaviour, and strategies for improving it in your child.

Step 4: Take Down Toxins explains the toxic mismatch we are in the modern world and how autistic children may struggle more to eliminate heavy metals from their bodies. We also discuss natural and non-invasive methods to support autistic children in detoxifying their bodies.

Step 5: Solve With Supplements explains which supplements you can purchase for your child to support their physical and brain health and the benefits of doing so.

Step 6: Charge the Cerebellum explains the role of the cerebellum in the brain, the tendency for autistic children to have a smaller cerebellum, and how parents can utilise neuroplasticity principles to promote the growth of their child's cerebellum.

Step 7: Empower Emotions aims to give parents practical ways to teach their child emotional literacy skills and explains the long-term benefits for your child of doing so.

The 7-Step Autism Action Plan aims to equip parents to know how to help their children, make the most of your child's early years intervention period, and unlock the potential of your autistic child to thrive in every way that they choose to.

It aims to empower parents to not need to rely on external experts who can ask you to sit tight for a few years to get an official diagnosis, and whose appointments can be so unreliable, or can be cancelled at any time if there is a staff strike or another pandemic. Instead you can take the control to make these simple changes for your child at home, to help your child meet their developmental milestones and unlock the potential you see inside of them.

The freedom from relying on external experts means you can create a calmer home environment sooner. Experience the joy of having a more emotionally regulated child, fostering their self-image and behaviour habits at a young age to thrive confidently in any environment.

Additionally, implementing my 7-Step Autism Action Plan has had another positive impact: My clients have shared that their other children feel more connected as siblings and no longer feel the need to assume a parental role for their autistic sibling.

A lot of my clients also feel like they have their lives back again, their sleep back again, and they can finally begin to make plans for their family how they imagined they would be able to.

With countless benefits for families, I encourage you to begin implementing the 7-Step Autism Action Plan today. Take control and start this journey today towards positive change.

After you've put the lifestyle changes suggested in this book into practice in the order recommended, it typically takes around 12 to 16 months to see a permanent turnaround in your child's autism. During this time, you'll likely observe a noticeable increase in your child's ability to learn new skills, helping them to reach their developmental milestones faster. Additionally, their physical health and immunity will often show an improvement as well.

I want to make it clear that your child may always be genetically vulnerable to developing autism symptoms again, through suffering a regression if these habits are not implemented continuously as a lifestyle change for you all. Also, if the child has a traumatic life event or an exposure to a toxin or an antibiotics prescription, this could trigger some of their autism symptoms reappearing as a regression too.

This is in line with epigenetics, which says that genes can be switched on and off depending on the environment. However, for all of my clients, once they see their child is thriving, has friends and is fitting in, this is motivation enough to continue these lifestyle recommendations for good.

To set yourself up for success, scan the QR code below to gain access to an invaluable e-bundle of resources, including at-home worksheets, child-friendly recipes, and tools designed to kickstart the implementation of the 7-Step Autism Action Plan for your child. This e-bundle is valued at £120 but with the Promo Code "Transform5" you are entitled to 20% off. Start your journey towards transformation today!

If you are interested in joining a group of similarly motivated parents on a structured program who are working on a common goal to unlock their autistic child's potential, then visit:

www.autismbrainempowerment.com to apply for my program. Working in a group of parents who all have similar goals means that you are 70% more likely to reach your goals and stay motivated on your journey, compared to people who work towards a goal individually.

In the world of parenting an autistic child, the power to effect change lies in the parents hands. The 7-Step Autism Action Plan is not just a set of instructions; it is a roadmap to unlocking your child's potential and guiding them toward reaching their developmental milestones with greater ease and speed.

So I invite you to take the first step today. Together we can achieve remarkable results and chart a course toward a brighter and easier tomorrow.

About the Author

Taiba Bajar is an award-winning researcher and licensed brain health trainer. With a seasoned background as a corporate professional and parent coach, she holds two science degrees from the University of Bristol with a background in neuroscience.

Taiba founded Autism Brain Empowerment™, a successful parent coaching business following her journey as a parent to her autistic son. Drawing from her professional expertise and personal experiences, Taiba equips parents to guide their children in reducing autism symptoms, unlocking their potential, and fostering their leadership in the world.

If you would like to stay in touch with Taiba, you can follow her on social media:

@autismbrainempowerment

taibabajar

Autism Brain Empowerment

@autismbrainempowerment

@AutismBrainEmpowerment

@AutismBrainEmUK

References

1. Jones, K. (2022) *Early childhood brain development has lifelong impact, Arizona PBS*. Available at: https://azpbs.org/2017/11/early-childhood-brain-development-lifelong-impact/ (Accessed: 12 February 2024).

2. Shana (2023) *3 Benefits of Neuroplasticity for Children with Autism, 3 benefits of neuroplasticity for children with autism*. Available at: https://www.re-origin.com/articles/neuroplasticity-children-with-autism (Accessed: 06 March 2024).

3. Castelbaum, L. *et al.* (2019) 'On the nature of monozygotic twin concordance and discordance for autistic trait severity: A quantitative analysis', *Behavior Genetics*, 50(4), pp. 263–272. doi:10.1007/s10519-019-09987-2.

4. Becker, H.S. (1997) *Outsiders: Studies in the sociology of deviance*. New York: Free Press.

5. Weinstock, C.P. (2022) *The deep emotional ties between depression and autism, Spectrum*. Available at: https://www.spectrumnews.org/features/deep-dive/the-deep-emotional-ties-between-depression-and-autism/ (Accessed: 06 March 2024).

6. Stanborough, R.J. (2021) *Understanding autism masking and its consequences, Healthline.* Available at: https://www.healthline.com/health/autism/autism-masking#stages (Accessed: 21 February 2024).

7. *Mitochondria: Form, function, and disease* (no date) *Medical News Today.* Available at: https://www.medicalnewstoday.com/articles/320875#function (Accessed: 12 February 2024).

8. Brand, M.D. *et al.* (2013) 'The role of mitochondrial function and cellular bioenergetics in ageing and disease', *British Journal of Dermatology,* 169, pp. 1–8. doi:10.1111/bjd.12208.

9. Zuryn, S. (2017) *Mitochondria: What are they and why do we have them?, Queensland Brain Institute - University of Queensland.* Available at: https://qbi.uq.edu.au/brain/brain-anatomy/mitochondria-what-are-they-and-why-do-we-have-them (Accessed: 06 March 2024).

10. *Unravelling mitochondria's mysterious link to autism* (2008) *Spectrum.* Available at: https://www.spectrumnews.org/news/unraveling-mitochondrias-mysterious-link-to-autism/ (Accessed: 12 February 2024).

11. Palmer, C.M. (2022) *Brain energy: A revolutionary breakthrough in understanding mental health--and improving treatment for anxiety, depression, OCD, PTSD, and more.* Dallas, TX: BenBella Books, Inc.

12. I would like to credit Dr Daniel Amen who has inspired this table below with his "killing the ANTS (automatic negative thoughts) technique.

13. Ito, E., Shima, R. and Yoshioka, T. (2019) 'A novel role of oxytocin: Oxytocin-induced well-being in humans', *Biophysics and Physicobiology*, 16(0), pp. 132–139. doi:10.2142/biophysico.16.0_132.

14. Lee, H.-J. *et al.* (2009) 'Oxytocin: The great facilitator of life', *Progress in Neurobiology* [Preprint]. doi:10.1016/j.pneurobio.2009.04.001.

15. Lee, H.-J. *et al.* (2009) 'Oxytocin: The great facilitator of life', *Progress in Neurobiology* [Preprint]. doi:10.1016/j.pneurobio.2009.04.001.

16. Yao, S. and Kendrick, K.M. (2022) 'Effects of intranasal administration of oxytocin and vasopressin on social cognition and potential routes and mechanisms of action', *Pharmaceutics*, 14(2), p. 323. doi:10.3390/pharmaceutics14020323.

17. Ford, C.L. and Young, L.J. (2021) 'Refining oxytocin therapy for autism: Context is key', *Nature Reviews Neurology*, 18(2), pp. 67–68. doi:10.1038/s41582-021-00602-9.

18. Harvey, A.R. (2020) 'Links between the neurobiology of oxytocin and human musicality', *Frontiers in Human Neuroscience*, 14. doi:10.3389/fnhum.2020.00350.

19. *Why reading nursery rhymes and singing to babies may help them to learn language* (2023) *University of Cambridge*. Available at: https://www.cam.ac.uk/research/news/why-reading-nursery-rhymes-and-singing-to-babies-may-help-them-to-learn-language (Accessed: 12 February 2024).

20. Harvey, A.R. (2020) 'Links between the neurobiology of oxytocin and human musicality', *Frontiers in Human Neuroscience*, 14. doi:10.3389/fnhum.2020.00350.

21. *Why reading nursery rhymes and singing to babies may help them to learn language* (2023) *University of Cambridge*. Available at: https://www.cam.ac.uk/research/news/why-reading-nursery-rhymes-and-singing-to-babies-may-help-them-to-learn-language (Accessed: 12 February 2024).

22. *Oxytocin: The love hormone* (2023) *Harvard Health*. Available at: https://www.health.harvard.edu/mind-and-mood/oxytocin-the-love-hormone#:~:text=Just%20the%20simple%20act

%20of,the%20four%20feel%2Dgood%20hormon es. (Accessed: 12 February 2024).

23. Rassovsky, Y. *et al.* (2019) 'Martial arts increase oxytocin production', *Scientific Reports*, 9(1). doi:10.1038/s41598-019-49620-0.

24. Ellingsen, D.-M. *et al.* (2016) 'The Neurobiology Shaping Affective Touch: Expectation, motivation, and meaning in the multisensory context', *Frontiers in Psychology*, 6. doi:10.3389/fpsyg.2015.01986.

25. Henderson, E.F. (2022) 'Autism, autonomy, and touch avoidance', *Disability Studies Quarterly*, 42(1). doi:10.18061/dsq.v42i1.7714.

26. Marshall-Pescini, S. *et al.* (2019) 'The role of oxytocin in the dog–owner relationship', *Animals*, 9(10), p. 792. doi:10.3390/ani9100792.

27. McCann, S., Perapoch Amadó, M. and Moore, S. (2020) 'The role of Iron in Brain Development: A Systematic Review', *Nutrients*, 12(7), p. 2001. doi:10.3390/nu12072001.

28. Pino, J.M. *et al.* (2017) 'Iron-restricted diet affects brain ferritin levels, dopamine metabolism and cellular prion protein in a region-specific manner', *Frontiers in Molecular Neuroscience*, 10. doi:10.3389/fnmol.2017.00145.

29. Juárez Olguín, H. *et al.* (2017) 'The role of dopamine and its dysfunction as a consequence of oxidative stress', *Oxidative Medicine and*

Cellular Longevity, 2017, pp. 1–13.
doi:10.1155/2016/9730467.

30. Mayo Clinic Staff (2022) *Iron deficiency anemia,*
    Mayo Clinic. Available at:
    https://www.mayoclinic.org/diseases-
    conditions/iron-deficiency-anemia/diagnosis-
    treatment/drc-20355040 (Accessed: 06 March
    2024).

31. Krigsman, A. and Walker, S.J. (2021)
    'Gastrointestinal disease in children with
    autism spectrum disorders: Etiology or
    consequence?', *World Journal of Psychiatry*, 11(9),
    pp. 605–618. doi:10.5498/wjp.v11.i9.605.

32. Nazem, M.R. *et al.* (2021) 'The relationship
    between thyroid function tests and sleep
    quality: cross-sectional study', *Journal of Sleep
    Science*, 14(3). doi:10.5498/wjp.v11.i9.605.

33. *Psychological symptoms and thyroid disorders*
    (2018) *British Thyroid Foundation*. Available at:
    https://www.btf-thyroid.org/psychological-
    symptoms-and-thyroid-disorders (Accessed: 06
    March 2024).

34. Pereira, H. (2017) 'The importance of
    cholesterol in psychopathology: A review of
    recent contributions', *Indian Journal of
    Psychological Medicine*, 39(2), pp. 109–113.
    doi:10.4103/0253-7176.203117.

35. Kępka, A. *et al.* (2021) 'Potential role of L-carnitine in autism spectrum disorder', *Journal of Clinical Medicine*, 10(6), p. 1202. doi:10.3390/jcm10061202.

36. Muskens, J. *et al.* (2022) 'Vitamin D status in children with a psychiatric diagnosis, autism spectrum disorders, or internalizing disorders', *Frontiers in Psychiatry*, 13. doi:10.3389/fpsyt.2022.958556.

37. Pedersen, T. (2023) *B12 and depression: What's the connection?*, *Psych Central*. Available at: https://psychcentral.com/depression/b12-and-depression (Accessed: 06 March 2024).

38. Parletta, N., Niyonsenga, T. and Duff, J. (2016) 'Omega-3 and omega-6 polyunsaturated fatty acid levels and correlations with symptoms in children with attention deficit hyperactivity disorder, autistic spectrum disorder and typically developing controls', *PLOS ONE*, 11(5). doi:10.1371/journal.pone.0156432.

39. Dighriri, I.M. *et al.* (2022) 'Effects of omega-3 polyunsaturated fatty acids on Brain Functions: A systematic review', *Cureus* [Preprint]. doi:10.7759/cureus.30091.

40. Christine Hammond, M. (2019) *The unfortunate connection between lyme disease and mental illness*, *Psych Central*. Available at: https://psychcentral.com/pro/exhausted-

woman/2019/07/the-unfortunate-connection-between-lyme-disease-and-mental-illness#1 (Accessed: 06 March 2024).

41. X, S. (2021) *A low omega-3 index is just as strong a predictor of early death as smoking, Medical Xpress - medical research advances and health news.* Available at: https://medicalxpress.com/news/2021-06-omega-index-strong-predictor-early.html (Accessed: 06 March 2024).

42. Ravalia, S. (2024). Cut Out The Bullshit: There's Always Another Way. London: Inspired by Publishing.

43. Ravalia, S. (2024). Cut Out The Bullshit: There's Always Another Way. London: Inspired by Publishing.

44. Thursby, E. and Juge, N. (2017) 'Introduction to the human gut microbiota', *Biochemical Journal,* 474(11), pp. 1823–1836. doi:10.1042/bcj20160510.

45. Zoe Ltd (no date) *The more the merrier. why diversity matters for your gut microbiome, Zoe.* Available at: https://zoe.com/post/gut-bacteria-diversity (Accessed: 06 March 2024).

46. Jandhyala, S.M. (2015) 'Role of the normal gut microbiota', *World Journal of Gastroenterology,* 21(29), p. 8787. doi:10.3748/wjg.v21.i29.8787.

47. Zoe Ltd (no date b) *What's your gut feeling? the connection between your gut microbiome and mental health, Zoe.* Available at: https://zoe.com/post/gut-health-mood (Accessed: 06 March 2024).

48. Communications, D.O. | M. (2021a) *Gut-brain connection in autism, Harvard Medical School.* Available at: https://hms.harvard.edu/news/gut-brain-connection-autism (Accessed: 12 February 2024).

49. Taniya, M.A. *et al.* (2022) 'Role of gut microbiome in autism spectrum disorder and its therapeutic regulation', *Frontiers in Cellular and Infection Microbiology*, 12. doi:10.3389/fcimb.2022.915701.

50. Fowlie, G., Cohen, N. and Ming, X. (2018) 'The perturbance of microbiome and gut-brain axis in autism spectrum disorders', *International Journal of Molecular Sciences*, 19(8), p. 2251. doi:10.3390/ijms19082251.

51. Holingue C., Newill C., Lee L.C., Pasricha P.J., Daniele Fallin M. Gastrointestinal Symptoms in Autism Spectrum Disorder: A Review of the Literature on Ascertainment and Prevalence. *Autism Res.* 2017;11:24–36. doi: 10.1002/aur.1854

52. Thulasi V., Steer R.A., Monteiro I.M., Ming X. Overall Severities of Gastrointestinal Symptoms in Pediatric Outpatients with and without Autism Spectrum Disorder. *Autism.* 2018 doi: 10.1177/1362361318757564

53. Chaidez V., Hansen R.L., Hertz-Picciotto I. Gastrointestinal Problems in Children with Autism, Developmental Delays or Typical Development. J. Autism Dev. Disord. 2013;44:1117–1127. doi: 10.1007/s10803-013-1973-x.

54. Patangia, D.V. *et al.* (2022) 'Impact of antibiotics on the human microbiome and consequences for host health', *MicrobiologyOpen*, 11(1). doi:10.1002/mbo3.1260.

55. Browne, A.J. *et al.* (2021) 'Global antibiotic consumption and usage in humans, 2000–18: A spatial modelling study', *The Lancet Planetary Health*, 5(12). doi:10.1016/s2542-5196(21)00280-1.

56. *What happens to the gut microbiome after taking antibiotics?* (no date) *The Scientist Magazine®.* Available at: https://www.the-scientist.com/news-opinion/what-happens-to-the-gut-microbiome-after-taking-antibiotics-69970 (Accessed: 12 February 2024).

57. Myers, A. (no date) The solution to candida overgrowth I didn't learn in medical school,

Amy Myers MD. Available at:
https://www.amymyersmd.com/article/soluti
on-candida-med-school (Accessed: 12 February
2024).

58. Eske, J. and Chavoustie, C.T. (2024) *Leaky gut
syndrome: What it is, symptoms, and treatments,
Medical News Today.* Available at:
https://www.medicalnewstoday.com/articles
/326117 (Accessed: 06 March 2024).

59. Satokari, R. (2020) 'High intake of sugar and the
balance between pro- and anti-inflammatory
gut bacteria', *Nutrients,* 12(5), p. 1348.
doi:10.3390/nu12051348.

60. Evennett-Watts, B. (2023) *How to spot ultra-
processed foods, according to Professor Tim Spector,
Good House Keeping.* Available at:
https://www.goodhousekeeping.com/uk/lifes
tyle/a45810816/professor-tim-spector-top-tip-
spotting-ultra-processed-foods/ (Accessed: 06
March 2024).

61. Aleman, R.S., Moncada, M. and Aryana, K.J.
(2023) 'Leaky gut and the ingredients that help
treat it: A Review', *Molecules,* 28(2), p. 619.
doi:10.3390/molecules28020619.

62. *Proton-pump inhibitors - harvard health
publications* (2021) *Harvard Health Publishing.*
Available at:
https://www.health.harvard.edu/newsletter_a

rticle/proton-pump-inhibitors (Accessed: 06 March 2024).

63. Kamionkowski, S. *et al.* (2021) 'The relationship between gastroesophageal reflux disease and autism spectrum disorder in adult patients in the United States', *Neurogastroenterology & Motility*, 34(7). doi:10.1111/nmo.14295.

64. Carpita, B. *et al.* (2022) 'Autism spectrum disorder and foetal alcohol spectrum disorder: A literature review', *Brain Sciences*, 12(6), p. 792. doi:10.3390/brainsci12060792.

65. Whiteley, P. et al, (2010), The Scan Brit randomised, controlled single-blind study of a gluten and casein-free dietary intervention for children with autism spectrum disorders, Nutritional Neuroscience, Vol. 13(2) pp. 87-100

66. Alamri, E.S. (2020) 'Efficacy of gluten- and casein-free diets on autism spectrum disorders in children', *Saudi Medical Journal*, 41(10), pp. 1041–1046. doi:10.15537/smj.2020.10.25308.

67. Fasano, A. (2012) 'Zonulin, regulation of tight junctions, and autoimmune diseases', *Annals of the New York Academy of Sciences*, 1258(1), pp. 25–33. doi:10.1111/j.1749-6632.2012.06538.x.

68. Anderson, J. (2023) *Gluten ataxia: When gluten attacks your brain, Verywell Health.* Available at: https://www.verywellhealth.com/what-is-

gluten-ataxia-562400 (Accessed: 21 February 2024).

69. Mearns, E. *et al.* (2019) 'Neurological manifestations of neuropathy and ataxia in celiac disease: A systematic review', *Nutrients*, 11(2), p. 380. doi:10.3390/nu11020380.

70. Jackson, J.R. *et al.* (2011) 'Neurologic and psychiatric manifestations of celiac disease and gluten sensitivity', *Psychiatric Quarterly*, 83(1), pp. 91–102. doi:10.1007/s11126-011-9186-y.

71. Pruimboom, L. and de Punder, K. (2015) 'The opioid effects of gluten exorphins: Asymptomatic celiac disease', *Journal of Health, Population and Nutrition*, 33(1). doi:10.1186/s41043-015-0032-y.

72. Woodford, K.B. (2021) 'Casomorphins and gliadorphins have diverse systemic effects spanning gut, brain and internal organs', International Journal of Environmental Research and Public Health, 18(15), p. 7911. doi:10.3390/ijerph18157911.

73. Malik TF, Panuganti KK. Lactose Intolerance. [Updated 2023 Apr 17]. In: StatPearls [Internet]. Treasure Island (FL): StatPearls Publishing; 2024 Jan- Available from: https://www.ncbi.nlm.nih.gov/books/NBK53 2285/.

74. Kiefte-de Jong JC, et al. Infant nutritional factors and functional constipation in childhood: the Generation R study. Am J Gastroenterol. 2 March 2010 [Epub ahead of print]

75. *Clinical nutrition: Nutritional medicine: Children's hope centre: San Diego* (no date) *Nutritional Medicine | Children's HOPE Center | San Diego*. Available at: https://childrenshopecenter.com/practice-areas/clinical-nutrition (Accessed: 13 February 2024).

76. Ramaekers, V. *et al.* (2007) 'Folate receptor autoimmunity and cerebral folate deficiency in low-functioning autism with neurological deficits', *Neuropediatrics*, 38(6), pp. 276–281. doi:10.1055/s-2008-1065354.

77. Dwiyanto, J., Hussain, M.H., Reidpath, D. *et al.* Ethnicity influences the gut microbiota of individuals sharing a geographical location: a cross-sectional study from a middle-income country. *Sci Rep* 11, 2618 (2021). https://doi.org/10.1038/s41598-021-82311-3

78. Amadi, C.N. *et al.* (2022) 'Association of autism with toxic metals: A systematic review of Case-Control Studies', *Pharmacology Biochemistry and Behavior*, 212, p. 173313. doi:10.1016/j.pbb.2021.173313.

79. Lee, D.-H. and Jacobs Jr, D.R. (2019) 'New approaches to cope with possible harms of low-dose environmental chemicals', *Journal of Epidemiology and Community Health*, 73(3), pp. 193–197. doi:10.1136/jech-2018-210920.

80. Ding, M. *et al.* (2023) 'Association between heavy metals exposure (cadmium, lead, arsenic, mercury) and Child autistic disorder: A systematic review and meta-analysis', *Frontiers in Pediatrics*, 11. doi:10.3389/fped.2023.1169733.

81. Ding, M. *et al.* (2023a) 'Association between heavy metals exposure (cadmium, lead, arsenic, mercury) and Child autistic disorder: A systematic review and meta-analysis', *Frontiers in Pediatrics*, 11. doi:10.3389/fped.2023.1169733.

82. Balali-Mood, M. *et al.* (2021) 'Toxic mechanisms of five heavy metals: Mercury, lead, chromium, Cadmium, and arsenic', *Frontiers in Pharmacology*, 12. doi:10.3389/fphar.2021.643972.

83. Balali-Mood, M. *et al.* (2021) 'Toxic mechanisms of five heavy metals: Mercury, lead, chromium, Cadmium, and arsenic', *Frontiers in Pharmacology*, 12. doi:10.3389/fphar.2021.643972.

84. Ragusa, A. *et al.* (2021) 'Plasticenta: First evidence of microplastics in human placenta',

Environment International, 146, p. 106274.
doi:10.1016/j.envint.2020.106274.

85. Ravalia, S. (2024). Cut Out The Bullshit: There's Always Another Way. London: Inspired by Publishing.

86. Deth, R. *et al.* (2010) 'Redox imbalance and the metabolic pathology of autism', *Developmental Neurotoxicology Research*, pp. 477–499. doi:10.1002/9780470917060.ch22.

87. Grayson, D.R. and Guidotti, A. (2016) 'Merging data from genetic and epigenetic approaches to better understand autistic spectrum disorder', *Epigenomics*, 8(1), pp. 85–104. doi:10.2217/epi.15.92.

88. Dualde, P. *et al.* (2021) 'Biomonitoring of phthalates, bisphenols and parabens in children: Exposure, predictors and risk assessment', *International Journal of Environmental Research and Public Health*, 18(17), p. 8909. doi:10.3390/ijerph18178909.

89. Braun, J.M., Sathyanarayana, S. and Hauser, R. (2013) 'Phthalate exposure and children's health', *Current Opinion in Pediatrics*, 25(2), pp. 247–254. doi:10.1097/mop.0b013e32835e1eb6.

90. Hlisníková, H. *et al.* (2020) 'Effects and mechanisms of phthalates' action on reproductive processes and Reproductive Health: A Literature Review', *International*

Journal of Environmental Research and Public Health, 17(18), p. 6811.
doi:10.3390/ijerph17186811.

91. Wang, Y. and Qian, H. (2021) 'Phthalates and their impacts on human health', *Healthcare*, 9(5), p. 603. doi:10.3390/healthcare9050603.

92. Yuka, F. de (2022) *The mobile app that scans your diet and cosmetics, Yuka*. Available at: https://yuka.io/en/ (Accessed: 13 February 2024).

93. *Dirty thinkers' choice awards 2023 - think dirty®* (2023) *Think Dirty® Shop Clean*. Available at: https://www.thinkdirtyapp.com/awards/how -it-works/ (Accessed: 25 February 2024).

94. Suglia, S.F. *et al.* (2008) 'Association between lung function and cognition among children in a prospective birth cohort study', *Psychosomatic Medicine*, 70(3), pp. 356–362. doi:10.1097/psy.0b013e3181656a5a.

95. *Are lead water pipes still a problem in the UK?* (no date) *The Water Professor*. Available at: https://thewaterprofessor.com/blogs/articles/ lead-pipes (Accessed: 13 February 2024).

96. Evlampidou, I. *et al.* (2020) 'Trihalomethanes in drinking water and bladder cancer burden in the European Union', *Environmental Health Perspectives*, 128(1). doi:10.1289/ehp4495.

97. *Filtration* (no date) *Water2.com*. Available at: https://water2.com/pages/filtration (Accessed: 13 February 2024).

98. Peatross, J. (2022) *Mold toxicity syndrome and autism spectrum disorder, WellnessPlus by Dr. Jess.* Available at: https://app.drjessmd.com/mold-toxicity-syndrome-and-autism-spectrum-disorder/ (Accessed: 13 February 2024).

99. Starnes, H.M. *et al.* (2022) 'A critical review and meta-analysis of impacts of per- and polyfluorinated substances on the brain and behaviour', *Frontiers in Toxicology*, 4. doi:10.3389/ftox.2022.881584.

100. Braun, J.M. and Hauser, R. (2011) 'Bisphenol A and children's health', *Current Opinion in Pediatrics*, 23(2), pp. 233–239. doi:10.1097/mop.0b013e3283445675.

101. Mughal, B.B., Fini, J.-B. and Demeneix, B.A. (2018) 'Thyroid-disrupting chemicals and Brain Development: An update', *Endocrine Connections*, 7(4). doi:10.1530/ec-18-0029.

102. Boat, T.F. (2015) *Prevalence of autism spectrum disorder, Mental Disorders and Disabilities Among Low-Income Children.* Available at: https://www.ncbi.nlm.nih.gov/books/NBK332896/ (Accessed: 13 February 2024).

103. Yolande Loftus, B. (2024) *Autism statistics you need to know in 2024, Autism Parenting Magazine.*

Available at:
https://www.autismparentingmagazine.com/
autism-statistics/ (Accessed: 13 February 2024).

104. Gressier, M. and Frost, G. (2021) 'Minor
changes in fibre intake in the UK population
between 2008/2009 and 2016/2017', *European
Journal of Clinical Nutrition*, 76(2), pp. 322–327.
doi:10.1038/s41430-021-00933-2.

105. Ravalia, S. (2024). Cut Out The Bullshit: There's
Always Another Way. London: Inspired by
Publishing.

106. Doaei, S. *et al.* (2021) 'The effect of omega-3
fatty acids supplementation on social and
behavioural disorders of children with autism:
A randomised clinical trial', *Pediatric
Endocrinology Diabetes and Metabolism*, 27(1), pp.
12–18. doi:10.5114/pedm.2020.101806.

107. *Autism and omega-3: How the brain is positively
impacted* (no date) *Transformations*. Available at:
https://www.transformationsnetwork.com/po
st/autism-and-omega-3-how-the-brain-is-
positively-impacted (Accessed: 13 February
2024).

108. Bda (2024) *Fibre, Home*. Available at:
https://www.bda.uk.com/resource/fibre.html
(Accessed: 06 March 2024).

109. Ayati, Z., Yang, G., Ayati, M.H. *et al.* Saffron for
mild cognitive impairment and dementia: a

systematic review and meta-analysis of
randomised clinical trials. *BMC Complement
Med Ther* 20, 333 (2020).
https://doi.org/10.1186/s12906-020-03102-3

110. Van Essen, D.C., Donahue, C.J. and Glasser,
M.F. (2018) 'Development and evolution of
cerebral and cerebellar cortex', *Brain, Behavior
and Evolution*, 91(3), pp. 158–169.
doi:10.1159/000489943.

111. Srinivasan, S.M., Cavagnino, D.T. and Bhat,
A.N. (2018) 'Effects of equine therapy on
individuals with autism spectrum disorder: A
systematic review', *Review Journal of Autism and
Developmental Disorders*, 5(2), pp. 156–175.
doi:10.1007/s40489-018-0130-z.

112. McGavin, D.G. (2014) *The incredible human hand
and foot, BBC News*. Available at:
https://www.bbc.co.uk/news/science-
environment-26224631 (Accessed: 07 March
2024).

113. Gordon, S. (2023) *Get grounded: How walking
barefoot can improve your health, Health*. Available
at: https://www.health.com/grounding-
7968373 (Accessed: 13 February 2024).

114. LeedsAutismServices (no date) *Got Those Happy
Feet: The Benefits of Walking Barefoot, Leeds
Autism Services*. Available at:
https://www.leedsautism.org.uk/Handlers/D

ownload.ashx?IDMF=783fbe25-7d43-48ad-807f-9f290863ac82 (Accessed: 13 February 2024).

115. Bremer, E., Crozier, M. and Lloyd, M. (2016) 'A systematic review of the behavioural outcomes following exercise interventions for children and youth with autism spectrum disorder', *Autism*, 20(8), pp. 899–915. doi:10.1177/1362361315616002.

116. Marzbani, H., Marateb, H. and Mansourian, M. (2016) 'Methodological note: Neurofeedback: A comprehensive review on system design, methodology and clinical applications', *Basic and Clinical Neuroscience Journal*, 7(2). doi:10.15412/j.bcn.03070208.

117. *What to expect* (2024) *BrainTrainUK*. Available at: https://braintrainuk.com/what-to-expect/ (Accessed: 13 February 2024).

Printed in Great Britain
by Amazon

43132437R00106